Autonomic Pharmacology

Autonomic Pharmacology

Experimental and Clinical Aspects

Michael D Day

B. Pharm, Ph.D., M.I.Biol., F.P.S.

Director of Biological Research, Pharmaceutical Division of Reckitt and Colman, Ltd., Hull; Formerly Reader in Pharmacology, University of Aston, and Senior Lecturer in Pharmacology, University Hospital and Medical School, Nottingham.

CHURCHILL LIVINGSTONE

EDINBURGH LONDON AND NEW YORK 1979

CHURCHILL LIVINGSTONE
Medical Division of Longman Group Limited

Distributed in the United States of America by
Longman Inc., 19 West 44th Street, New York,
N.Y. 10036 and by associated companies, branches
and representatives throughout the world.

First Published 1979.

ISBN 0 443 01790 5

British Library Cataloguing in Publication Data
Day, Michael D
 Autonomic pharmacology.
 1. Autonomic drugs
 2. Nervous system, Autonomic
 I. Title
 615'.78   RM323   78–40708

Printed in Singapore by Huntsmen Offset Printing Pte Ltd

Preface

My principal justification for writing a book concerned with a single area of pharmacology is that my own teaching experience has taught me that autonomic pharmacology is often a topic which undergraduate students of medical science find confusing. At worst the subject may appear to consist of a seemingly endless list of drugs acting upon a variety of oddly-named receptor types and sub-types. The subject is not helped by a confusing and often illogical terminology which is compounded by some irritating differences between the terminology used in this country and that of the USA. My aims in this monograph have been to present the elements of the subject in what I hope is a simple style and using a consistent and logical terminology. I have tried to place each group of drugs into their respective historical contexts and to indicate how experimental pharmacology has led to the present level of understanding of drug action in man.

Our detailed knowledge of the functioning of the peripheral autonomic nervous system has progressed rapidly in the last thirty years and this has been greatly aided by the use of both new and existing drugs. For instance, the classic experiments of J. H. Burn and M. J. Rand which began in the late 1950's, uncovered many new facts concerning noradrenergic neuronal function by the skilful use of reserpine, itself an ancient therapeutic agent, as a pharmacological tool. Conversely, new drugs modifying autonomic nerve function and introduced in the last twenty years or so have had profound consequences for the treatment of serious illnesses such as hypertension and asthma which afflict mankind.

This book is intended primarily for undergraduate students of medical science and is broadly based on lecture courses I have delivered to students of Pharmacy and Medicine. I hope it will also be found useful to others such as post-graduate students who may wish to gain a grounding in what is a large and complex subject. For those who need to go deeper into any aspect of the subject I hope the references provided will at least serve as a useful starting point. I have included rather more information on clinical uses, dosage, preparations and trade-names than is usual in a text-book of pharmacology. I have done this deliberately since I wished to be as comprehensive as possible, and secondly, because I believe that many students are interested in this information even if it may not be immediately applicable to their formal examinations in pharmacology. I hope the information on drug dosage forms will also help students to distinguish between drugs which are mainly of pharmacological interest from those which are additionally of clinical importance.

I am grateful to many people who have helped me in various ways in the preparation of this book. In particular I should like to acknowledge the help of my former colleagues at Nottingham University Medical School; Miss Janet Mawby, Medical Librarian, Messrs. Geoff Lyth and Andrew Bezear, Medical Artists, and Mr. John Watson photographer. I am grateful to the editors of the journals indicated in the text and to various authors for allowing me to reproduce a number of figures from previously published scientific papers. I am indebted to many pharmaceutical companies for supplying me with much useful data regarding their drugs. Finally, I should like to thank my wife Marion for much patience and for typing successive drafts of the manuscript.

1979   M. D. D.

Contents

1

Discovery and general arrangement of the autonomic nervous system

The autonomic nervous system comprises those nervous elements whose function in the body is to regulate the activity of the mass of smooth muscle (also called unstriated or involuntary muscle) which is present largely in the hollow viscera of the body such as the gastrointestinal and respiratory tracts. In addition the autonomic nervous system innervates the cardiovascular system, the exocrine glandular ducts, smooth muscle containing structures in the eye such as the pupil and ciliary muscle and the pilomotor muscles of the skin.

The functioning of the autonomic nervous system is largely independent of conscious thought, the word autonomic being derived from the Greek autos (self) and nomos (law or governing). The relative independence of the autonomic nervous system comprises a valuable evolutionary asset for higher animals such as man since it allows of the maintenance of a relatively stable internal environment to the body, by controlling such vital functions as blood-perfusion of tissues and maintenance of a constant body temperature, without undue distraction of the more outward-looking higher brain centres. This ability to maintain constancy of bodily internal environment was aptly called *homeostasis* by W. B. Cannon (1929). The role of the autonomic nervous system in regulating the activity of smooth muscle is very different from that of the somatic system which controls the activity of striated muscle (also called voluntary or skeletal muscle). Striated muscle is almost totally dependent for its useful functioning on its innervation by somatic nerves. If the somatic nerve fibres innervating a skeletal muscle are destroyed then not only is the muscle paralysed but in time the muscle fibres weaken, become smaller and the muscle is said to atrophy. Smooth muscle on the other hand is not so dependent on its innervation, it does not atrophy when deprived of its extrinsic nerve supply and may in fact regain a good deal of its normal function after denervation. The reason for this is that smooth muscle cells are much less specialised than striated muscle cells and behave more like independent organisms.

Bozler (1948) classified vertebrate smooth muscle into two main types which he called single unit and multi-unit.

Single-unit smooth muscles include those of the gastro-intestinal tract and the uterus. These muscles characteristically show continuous rhythmic contractions and relaxations which are not dependent on any tonic influence from the autonomic nerves and are therefore termed *myogenic* (arising from the muscle). Although not dependent on nervous influences the myogenic activity may be modified (increased or decreased) by stimulation of autonomic nerves. In this type of smooth muscle there are junctions between the cells which facilitate the spread of conduction from one cell to another and allows activity to spread from an area of excitation to surrounding regions. Cardiac muscle is a structurally-modified form of smooth muscle and is a good example of this type of arrangement. Structures called intercalated discs occur between cardiac muscle cells and help in the rapid spread of excitation across the heart. The pumping action of the heart can be dramatically increased or decreased by stimulation of the appropriate extrinsic autonomic nerves whilst on the other hand it can continue to function quite well after all autonomic nerve influences have been abolished by drugs.

Multi-unit smooth muscles include the radial and ciliary muscle of the eye, the pilomotor muscles of the skin and the muscle in some blood vessels. Such muscles usually only con-tract in response to stimulation of their autonomic nerves, there appears to be no conduction between muscle cells and each cell is separately innervated.

In practice smooth muscles cannot be rigidly classified into one or other type and many behave as though intermediate between the two types. The speed of contraction of smooth muscle cells is very slow compared with skeletal muscle cells and the duration of contraction is often prolonged. The prolonged contraction of smooth muscle is often referred to as tone and may be dependent on the continuous arrival of nerve impulses (neuro-genic) or be due to spontaneous contraction of the smooth muscle (myogenic).

DISCOVERY OF THE AUTONOMIC NERVOUS SYSTEM

It was Galen the Greek physician of the second century AD who first clearly described structures which we now recognise as nerve trunks and ganglia of the autonomic nervous system. He suggested that there was 'sympathy' or 'consent' between different parts of the body and that this was brought about by the passage of 'animal spirits' through the nerves which he considered to be hollow tubes. According to Galen the vagi and sympathetic trunks were both functionally and anatomically a single unit. Most of Galen's teachings remained virtually unchallenged until 1545 when Estienne recognised that the sympathetic trunks and vagi were distinct anatomical structures. In 1664 Willis described accurately the course of the vagus ('Wanderer') nerve and made the very important distinction between voluntary and involuntary movements. Major contributions to our understanding of the functioning of the autonomic nervous system were made in the middle of the eighteenth century by Whytt. In 1751 he made the first allusion to autonomic reflex nervous activity when he suggested that involuntary movements were initiated by local stimulation due to nerve irritation and cited the peristaltic movements of the alimentary tract and the reaction of the pupil to light as examples. These brilliantly far-sighted suggestions were followed by another conceptual leap forward when he suggested (Whytt, 1765) that all 'sympathy' must be referred to the central nervous system since it occurred between parts of the body whose nerves were clearly not directly connected to each other. The word 'sympathetic' to describe a particular autonomic nerve was first applied by the Danish anatomist Winslow (1732) to the paravertebral sympathetic chains.

The nineteenth century saw the refinement of the microscope and of staining techniques and with them the emergence of histology as a branch of scientific investigation. Ehrenberg (1833) described cell bodies in sympathetic and spinal ganglia and this was followed by descriptions of the submucous plexus of the intestinal tract (Meissner, 1857) and the myenteric plexus (Auerbach, 1864). In 1834 Müller had described two kinds of muscle cell which he called striated and non-striated.

By the middle of the nineteenth century experimental physiology had developed as a separate scientific discipline largely due to the influence of the great French physiologist Claude Bernard. In 1851 Bernard clearly demonstrated the vasoconstrictor function of some sympathetic nerves. Our present day view of the structure and functioning of the autonomic nervous system we owe largely to two workers, the anatomist W. H. Gaskell, whose published work began in 1885 and is summarised in his book of 1916, and the Cambridge physiologist W. N. Langley. It was Langley who suggested the word 'autonomic' in place of 'involuntary' (which had been used by Gaskell) and further suggested the sub-division of the autonomic nervous system into sympathetic and parasympathetic systems.

GENERAL ANATOMY OF THE AUTONOMIC NERVOUS SYSTEM

The autonomic nervous system comprises a central portion lying within the central nervous system and a peripheral portion which is outside of the brain and spinal cord. The main centres of the brain involved in the regulation of autonomic activity are situated in the hypothalamus and in the medulla oblongata (hindbrain). Tracts of efferent fibres descend from the hypothalamus to form synapses with groups of cell bodies of medullary neurones and also with other cell bodies of neurones present in the lateral horns of the grey matter in the spinal cord. These medullary and spinal cord neurones send out efferent fibres (axons) which emerge from the central nervous system to synapse with the cell bodies of the final (excitor) neurones whose efferent axons innervate smooth muscle and glandular tissue. The cell bodies of the excitor neurones usually occur in clusters called ganglia (more correctly *autonomic ganglia*).

It should be stressed that although many autonomic functions occur without conscious thought and are therefore largely under hypothalamic and/or medullary control it is nevertheless clear that higher brain centres such as the cortex can profoundly effect autonomic activity. This is well illustrated by the case of the nervous student awaiting a *viva voce* examination. The apprehension occasioned by thoughts of the forthcoming ordeal may activate autonomic nerves supplying the sweat glands of the skin ('cold sweats'), the cardiovascular system (raised blood pressure and heart-rate), structures in the eyes (dilated pupils) and even, and perhaps most inconveniently, the bladder (desire to micturate). Langley who, on the suggestion of a colleague, coined the word autonomic in 1898 realised that the name might imply a greater degree of independence from the central nervous system than actually exists. He later wrote when referring to this problem '. . . it is, I think, more important that new words should be used for new ideas than that the words should be accurately descriptive'. (Langley, 1921).

It has been known for many years by students of yoga and

transcendental meditation that internal body functions can be profoundly altered by concentration and training. Research is in progress to try and use similar techniques to treat conditions such as anxiety and hypertension in which disfunction of central autonomic areas may play a part. Little is known at present of the physiology of the neural connections between higher and lower brain centres.

Our understanding of the functioning of the autonomic nervous system has been greatly simplified by the work of the anatomist W. H. Gaskell whose classic book summarising many of his findings was published posthumously in 1916. Langdon Brown paid tribute to Gaskell's work on the sympathetic system by writing in 1923;—'to read an account of the sympathetic nervous system before Gaskell is like reading a description of the circulation before Harvey'.

Gaskell recognised that much autonomic activity was reflexly initiated and that it was profitable to study the autonomic system in terms of reflex arcs since the same basic neural elements are involved in autonomic reflexes controlling smooth muscle activity as in somatic reflexes which control striated muscle activity. In a simple somatic reflex arc three neurones are typically involved (see Fig. 1.1):

1. The sensory (also called afferent or receptor) neurone with its endings, for instance, sensitive to heat and present in the skin with its cell body in the dorsal root ganglion or its cranial equivalent.
The axons of this neurone synapse with:
2. A connector (also called internuncial or interneurone) neurone in the dorsal horn of the grey matter which via its axon transmits the impulse to the ventral horn where it synapses with the cell body of:
3. The ventral horn cell and its axon which is called the motor or excitor neurone and which transmits efferent impulses to striated muscle. The autonomic reflex may be considered to be a variant of this. The sensory neurones appear to be similar in structure and function in both somatic and autonomic systems. However, in the autonomic reflex the sensory neurone synapses with the connector cell body somewhat deeper in the cord usually in the lateral horn of the grey matter (see Fig. 1.1). The major difference between somatic and autonomic reflexes is that in the autonomic reflex the axons from the connector neurones emerge from the spinal cord to synapse with the cell bodies (in

the autonomic ganglia) as the excitor neurones whose axons innervate the effector tissues. The part of the connector fibres emerging from the spinal cord and synapsing with the autonomic ganglia were called by Langley *preganglionic fibres* and those axons leaving the ganglia and synapsing finally with the effector tissues he called *postganglionic fibres*. By convention, and presumably because of the similarity between somatic and autonomic sensory neurones, the term autonomic nervous system is used to include only the efferent neurones supplying the viscera, i.e. the connector and excitor neurones.

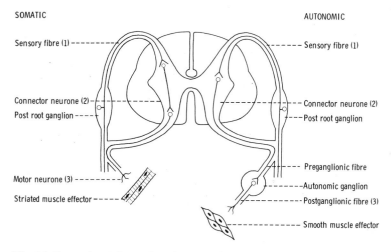

SOMATIC   AUTONOMIC

Sensory fibre (1) ------   ------ Sensory fibre (1)

Connector neurone (2) -   ------ Connector neurone (2)
Post root ganglion ----   ----Post root ganglion

                                             --- Preganglionic fibre
Motor neurone (3) --------   -------Autonomic ganglion
Striated muscle effector -----   ----------Postganglionic fibre (3)

                                             -------- Smooth muscle effector

Fig. 1.1 Comparison of somatic and autonomic reflex arcs (modified from Gaskell, 1916). Each arc consists of the same three basic neuronal components: (1) Sensory (afferent) neurones with cell bodies in posterior root ganglia synapse with connector neurones (2) in dorsal horn of grey matter (somatic) or in the lateral horn (autonomic). In the somatic system the connector neurones (2) remain within the grey matter and synapse in the ventral horn with the cell bodies of the somatic motorneurone (3) fibres from which emerge from the cord to innervate striated muscle. In the autonomic system the connector cell fibres emerge from the cord as preganglionic fibres to synapse in the autonomic ganglia with the cell bodies of the final neurones (3). The postganglionic fibres emerging from the autonomic ganglia innervate smooth muscle effectors.

There are differences in the nature of the axons involved in somatic and autonomic reflexes. The motor fibres of the somatic system are medullated (i.e. have a myelin sheath), have a diameter in the range 1–20μ and are termed A fibres. The preganglionic fibres of the autonomic system are also medullated but, in general, they are of smaller diameter being mostly in the range 1–3μ; they are called B fibres. C fibres are non-medullated, are generally under 1μ in diameter and include all postganglionic fibres of the autonomic system. Since the speed of conduction in nerve fibres is inversely proportional to the fibre diameter it follows that conduction in A fibres of the somatic system is much more rapid than in B and C fibres of the autonomic system.

The largest A fibres (20μ diameter) conduct impulses at a rate of approximately 120 metres/sec whilst C fibres of 1μ diameter conduct at only about 5 metres/sec.

SUBDIVISIONS OF THE AUTONOMIC NERVOUS SYSTEM

The autonomic nervous system, largely as a result of the work of Gaskell and Langley, has been subdivided into *sympathetic* and *parasympathetic* systems. This division was made originally on the grounds of the anatomical work of Gaskell but was subsequently substantiated by the physiological and pharmacological studies of Langley and of many later workers. Anatomically, the sympathetic division consists of the preganglionic fibres arising from the *thoracic* and *lumbar* regions of the spinal cord together with the peripheral ganglia with which they synapse and the postganglionic axons associated with them. The parasympathetic division consists of preganglionic fibres from the *medulla oblongata* and the *sacral* region of the cord together with their respective ganglia and postganglionic axons.

The sympathetic system. Preganglionic sympathetic fibres pass from the spinal cord with the anterior roots and leave the vertebral column with the segmental spinal nerves. They branch off from the spinal nerves as myelinated trunks (*white rami communicantes*) and join the chain of sympathetic ganglia (*paravertebral sympathetic chains*) which are situated on either side of the vertebral column. The preganglionic fibres of the sympathetic nervous system terminate in two main ways with the cell bodies of the excitor neurones (see Fig. 1.2). Firstly, they may synapse within the vertebral ganglion adjacent to the segment of the cord from which they left. However, many preganglionic fibres branch and may course up or down the cord to synapse within vertebral ganglia at some distance from their own point of exit from the cord. The postganglionic axons of the sympathetic ganglia may exit from the paravertebral ganglia either as postganglionic nerve trunks or they may pass back to the same segmental spinal nerve which contributed the white ramus to the ganglion in which case they are known as *grey rami communicantes* and the postganglionic axons ultimately branch off from the spinal nerves and travel to the effector tissues. The second main way in which preganglionic sympathetic fibres synapse is by passing through the sympathetic chains and synapsing with peripherally situated (sometimes called *prevertebral*) ganglia which lie in the abdominal cavity. Important

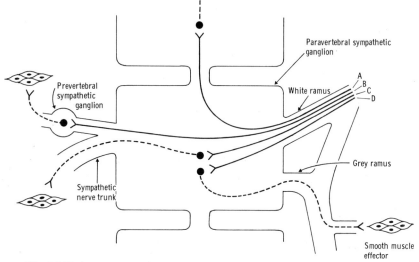

Fig. 1.2 Various courses which may be taken by preganglionic sympathetic fibres (solid lines) emerging from a spinal segment as a white ramus. Postganglionic fibres are shown as broken lines. Fibre A passes through the adjacent paravertebral ganglion and synapses within another paravertebral ganglion. Fibre B passes through the adjacent paravertebral ganglion to synapse with a prevertebral ganglion in the abdominal cavity. Fibre C synapses within the adjacent paravertebral ganglion and postganglionic fibres leave the ganglion as a sympathetic trunk. Fibre D synapses within the adjacent paravertebral ganglion and the postganglionic fibres pass back (in the grey ramus) to the same segmental nerve which contributed the white ramus. (Modified from Rand, Raper & McCulloch, 1971).

examples of these are the coeliac and mesenteric ganglia. Additionally, some preganglionic fibres pass through the sympathetic chains without synapsing and directly innervate the cells of the medullae of the adrenal glands. The adrenal glands are situated in the abdominal cavity close to the kidneys and the medullary portions are derived embryonically from the same tissue as postganglionic sympathetic neurones. It is convenient to think of the adrenal medullae as modified sympathetic ganglia and they have an important role in the body to re-inforce the action of the sympathetic system.

The parasympathetic system. The preganglionic axons of the parasympathetic system do not synapse within ganglia close to the vertebral column instead they synapse within ganglia which are usually very close to, or more often actually in, the effector organ. Often the cell bodies of the excitor neurones are diffusely distributed within a tissue, as for example in the gastrointestinal tract where they lie in the myenteric (Auerbach's) plexus, and thus no discrete ganglia, as occur in the sympathetic system, are visible. The postganglionic axons arising from parasympathetic ganglia are very short, branched processes which like sympathetic postganglionic axons are non-myelinated. The anatomical arrangement of parasympathetic ganglia and their postganglionic processes has made them technically difficult to study experimentally and as a consequence much less is known of their physiology than is the case with analogous structures in the sympathetic system.

SUMMARY

The autonomic nervous system modifies the activity of smooth and cardiac muscle and influences the secretion of some glandular tissue. It has a major role in higher animals in the maintenance of homeostasis. The autonomic system is controlled, largely subconsciously, from mid and hind-brain regions and is divided into sympathetic and parasympathetic systems. This division was made originally on anatomical grounds and has been largely substantiated by later physiological studies. When looked upon in terms of reflex arcs, the autonomic reflex contains the same basic neural elements as a somatic reflex: (1) a sensory (afferent) neurone (2) a connector neurone and (3) an excitor (motor neurone). The main anatomical difference in the two systems lies in the position of the connector neurones which remain in the grey matter of the spinal cord in the somatic reflex but emerge as preganglionic fibres to synapse with the cell bodies of excitor neurones in the autonomic system. Congregations of the cell bodies of the excitor neurones are known as autonomic ganglia and the fibres arising from them as postganglionic fibres. Sympathetic ganglia are mostly situated in the paravertebral ganglionic chains with some prevertebral ganglia present in the abdomen and, in general, have short myelinated preganglionic fibres and long unmyelinated postganglionic fibres. Parasympathetic ganglia are usually more diffusely arranged in, or very close to, the tissue innervated and have long myelinated preganglionic fibres and short unmyelinated postganglionic fibres.

REFERENCES

Auerbach, L. (1864) Fernere vorläufige mittheilung über den nervenapparat des darmes, *Virchows Arch. path. Anat.* **30**, 457–460.

Bernard, C. (1851) Influence du grand sympathique sur la sensibilité et sur la calorification, *C.r. Séanc. Soc. Biol.* **3**, 163–164.

Bozler, E. (1948) Conduction, automaticity, and tonus of visceral muscles. *Experientia*, **4**, 213–218.

Cannon, W. B. (1929) Organisation for physiological homeostasis. *Physiol. Rev.*, **9**, 399–431.

Ehrenberg, C. G. (1833) Nothwendigkeit einer feineren mechanischen zerlegung des gehirns und der nerven vor der chemischen, dargestellt aus Beobachtungen. *Ann. d. Phys. u. Chem.*, **28**, 449–472.

Estienne, S. C. (1545) *De Dissectione Partium Corporis Humani*. Paris: S. Colins.

Galen, C. (1854) De usu partium corporis humani, vol. 9, chap. 11. In *Oeuvres Anatomiques Physiologiques et Médicales de Galien*, vol. 1, translated by C. Daremberg. Paris: J. B. Bailliere.

Langdon Brown, W. (1923) *The Sympathetic Nervous System in Disease*. 2nd edn, London: Henry Frowde, and Hodder and Stoughton.

Langley, J. N. (1898) On the union of cranial autonomic (visceral) fibres with the nerve cells of the superior cervical ganglion. *J. Physiol.*, **23**, 240–270.

Meissner, G. (1857) Ueber die nerven der darmwand, *Ztschr. f. rat. Med.* **8**, 364–366.

Müller, J. (1834) *Handbuch der Physiologie des Menschen für Vorlesungen*, Coblenz, J. Hölscher, translated by Baly, W. London: Taylor & Walton, 1840.

Rand, M. J., Raper, C. & McCulloch, M. W. (1971) *Physiology and Pharmacology of the Autonomic Nervous System*, 2nd Impression. Melbourne: Australasian Pharmaceutical Publishing Co. Ltd.

Whytt, R. (1751) *An Essay on the Vital and Other Involuntary Motions of Animals*, Edinburgh: Hamilton, Balfour & Neill.

Whytt, R. (1765) *Observations on the Nature, Causes, and Cure of Those Disorders Which Have Been Commonly Called Nervous, Hypochondriac or Hysteric; To Which Are Prefixed Some Remarks on the Sympathy of the Nerves*, 2nd edn. Edinburgh: T. Beckett.

Willis, T. (1664) *Cerebri Anatome, Cui Accessit Nervorum Descriptio et Usus*, London: J. Flesher.

Winslow, J. B. (1732) *Exposition Anatomique de la Structure du Corps Humain*, Paris: G. Desprez; English translation by Douglas, G. London: A. Bettsworth and C. Hitch, 1734.

GENERAL READING

Gaskell, W. H. (1916) *The Involuntary Nervous System*, London: Longmans, Green & Co.

Kuntz, A. (1953) *The Autonomic Nervous System*, 4th edn. Philadelphia: Lee & Febiger.

Langley, J. N. (1921) *The Autonomic Nervous System*, Cambridge: W. Heffer & Sons Ltd.

Pick, J. (1970) *The Autonomic Nervous System*, Chapter 1. pp 3–21, Philadelphia: J. B. Lippincott Company.

Samson Wright's *Applied Physiology*, twelfth edition revised by C. A. Keele & E. Neil (1971) London: Oxford University Press.

Sheehan, D. (1936) Discovery of the autonomic nervous system. *Arch. Neurol Psychiat.*, **35**, 1081–1115.

2

Anatomy and physiology of the autonomic nervous system

The classification of the autonomic nervous system into sympathetic and parasympathetic divisions was made on both anatomical and physiological grounds. Gaskell (1886) noting that many tissues received fibres from both divisions suggested that the innervation was reciprocal or antagonistic. In some organs such as the eye and heart the antagonistic nature of sympathetic and parasympathetic innervations is well illustrated. However, in other tissues it is much less clear, some tissues receiving fibres from only one branch of the autonomic system whilst in others the two systems may produce similar or unrelated effects.

To generalise, the sympathetic system is concerned with preparing the body for increased activity whilst the parasympathetic has a conserving effect on bodily resources. The American physiologist W. B. Cannon described the effects of extreme sympathetic activation as preparing the body for flight or fight. In such a situation of profound fear or excitement the heart-rate and force of contraction are increased and hence blood flow to the skeletal muscles is increased, the muscle of the respiratory tract is relaxed facilitating passage of air into the lungs; the pupils are dilated, blood glucose level increased and the bodily hair is erected. Simultaneously, functions such as digestion, which are not immediately essential for survival, are suppressed. The parasympathetic system has less spectacular, but equally important, functions such as involvement in digestion, sweating, defaecation and micturation. In general, sympathetic activation leads to more widespread effects than does parasympathetic activation and this is reflected in the anatomy of the sympathetic innervation of many tissues. Sympathetic postganglionic fibres serving a particular tissue often arise from a number of different ganglia and there is much branching of preganglionic fibres in the sympathetic chains and elsewhere leading to synaptic connections being made with ganglion cells at varying sites and thus to much overlapping of innervations. Thus it is often difficult to state precisely the source of all of the nerve fibres, particularly sympathetic, supplying a particular tissue and text-books differ considerably in the details given of autonomic innervation. The situation is further complicated both by species differences and by variations between human individuals. In the account that follows the major known sources in man of both sympathetic and parasympathetic nerves are given and a somewhat simplified summary is illustrated in Fig. 2.1. It is likely that the system in its finest detail is much more complex. (See front flap for coloured version of Fig. 2.1.)

INNERVATION OF TISSUES BY THE AUTONOMIC NERVOUS SYSTEM AND THE EFFECTS PRODUCED BY AUTONOMIC ACTIVITY

Head and neck region
The connector cells supplying sympathetic fibres to structures in this region arise from the lateral horns of the upper three thoracic segments (T1 to T3) of the spinal cord. They pass to the paravertebral sympathetic chains and synapse in the superior cervical ganglion with the cell bodies of the excitor neurones. The postganglionic fibres arising from the superior cervical ganglion pass to the various tissues innervated in this area.

The eye
Postganglionic sympathetic nerve fibres terminate in the radial smooth muscle of the pupil (*dilator pupilloe muscle*) and in the smooth muscle present in the upper and lower eyelids (superior and inferior tarsal muscles respectively) and in the blood vessels of the conjunctiva and retina. The parasympathetic nerves to the eye arise from the Edinger-Westphal nucleus in the midbrain and pass via the oculomotor (IIIrd cranial) nerve to the ciliary ganglion where they synapse with the cell bodies of the excitor neurones. The postganglionic fibres arising from the ciliary ganglion innervate the circular muscle of the iris (*constrictor pupilloe muscle*) and the smooth muscle of the ciliary body.

Effects of autonomic stimulation. Sympathetic stimulation causes dilatation of the pupil (*mydriasis*) accompanied by retraction of the eyelids, especially the upper lid, producing a 'staring' gaze. The blood vessels of the conjunctiva and retina are constricted. Parasympathetic stimulation contracts the circular (concentrically-arranged) muscle of the iris and therefore reduces the diameter of the pupil (*miosis*). Parasympathetic activity also contracts the ciliary body thus altering the tension on the suspensory ligaments which in turn alter the tension on, and therefore curvature of, the lens. When the smooth muscle of the ciliary body is relaxed the suspensory ligaments hold the lens under tension, its curvature is decreased and it is focussed for distant objects. When the ciliary body contracts under parasympathetic influence, it is pulled forward, lessening the tension on the lens produced by the suspensory ligaments and allowing the lens to assume a greater curvature and focussing it for near vision. This process is called *accommodation* and in practice when the eyes are focussed from a distant to a near object there occurs a simultaneous constriction of the pupil by parasympathetic influence which produces an increased resolving power of the lens. In man, changes in pupil diameter are normally produced by alterations in parasympathetic activity, the sympathetic having relatively little effect. However, a sympathetically-induced mydriasis may occur in emotional states such as fear and rage.

The movements of the ciliary body and the iris in response to parasympathetic stimulation result in an increase in the angle between the anterior surface of the iris and the internal surface of the cornea (*filtration angle*) and this facilitates penetration of aqueous humour into the canal of Schlemm from which it is drained into the lymphatic system.

The lachrymal glands
The lachrymal glands receive postganglionic sympathetic fibres from the superior cervical ganglion. The parasympathetic supply leaves the brain stem in the facial (VIIth cranial) nerve which synapses with the sphenopalatine ganglion from which arise the postganglionic fibres which innervate the glandular cells. The sympathetic nerves mainly innervate the blood vessels of the gland and produce vasoconstriction; they may also, to a lesser extent, stimulate tear production. Parasympathetic stimulation markedly increases tear production.

The salivary glands
The salivary glands receive sympathetic postganglionic fibres arising from the superior cervical ganglion and which end mainly in the blood vessels of the glands. However, there may be, in addition, some direct sympathetic innervation of mucous cells.

The parasympathetic supply arises from the brain-stem and travels to the glands via the facial (VIIth cranial) and glosso-pharyngeal (IXth) nerves which synapse in the submandibular and otic ganglia respectively. The *submandibular* and *sublingual* salivary glands receive postganglionic fibres from the sub-mandibular ganglion and the *parotid* gland from the otic gang-lion.

Effects of autonomic stimulation. Some authorities consider that sympathetic stimulation evokes the secretion of thick saliva containing many cells. However, it is not clear whether this is a direct effect of the sympathetic system on secretory cells or whether it is a secondary change due to reduction in blood flow through the glands caused by sympathetic vasoconstriction. Parasympathetic stimulation causes the secretion of thin watery saliva and this system is clearly of greater importance in the normal functioning of the glands.

The pituitary gland
The pituitary gland receives sympathetic postganglionic fibres from the superior cervical ganglion the majority of which end in the anterior lobe and the remainder in the posterior lobe. Para-sympathetic fibres arise in the supraoptic and paraventricular hypothalamic nuclei and end mostly in the posterior lobe with only a few fibres ending in the pars intermedia and anterior lobe. The secretory mechanisms of the pituitary are of great com-plexity and clearly depend to a great extent on hormonal activity. However, there is evidence to suggest that some pituitary secretions are initiated through autonomic influence although the details are as yet unclear.

Blood vessels of the head
Sympathetic postganglionic fibres arise mainly from the superior cervical ganglia with their connector cells mostly arising from the upper two thoracic segments but with a smaller and variable contribution of preganglionic fibres from lower thoracic segments. Some blood vessels in the head such as the cerebral vessels and those supplying the mucous membranes of the mouth, nose and palate also receive a parasympathetic supply from the cranial parasympathetic nerves. Sympathetic stimulation causes vaso-constriction whilst parasympathetic fibres have a vasodilator function.

Organs of the skin
The skin in all parts of the body receives sympathetic post-ganglionic fibres usually from the adjacent ganglia in the sympathetic chains. In the head the sympathetic postganglionic fibres arise from the superior cervical ganglia and innervate the blood vessels of the skin, the sweat glands and the pilomotor muscles. The sweat glands in man are of two types; the *eccrine* glands which are widely distributed over the skin of the body and secrete dilute sweat in response to stimulation of the sympathetic fibres which innervate them and the *apocrine* glands which are larger and distributed mainly in the arm-pits and around the external genitalia. The apocrine glands are not innervated but are able to respond to catecholamines released by the adrenal medullae to increase secretion of sweat having a marked and characteristic odour.

Effects of autonomic stimulation. Sympathetic stimulation usually causes vasoconstriction of skin vessels although in some regions, such as the skin of the face, it produces vasodilatation as in the phenomenon of blushing. The pilomotor muscles which are attached to the hair follicle are contracted causing the follicles to stand out from the skin (*piloerection*). This mechanism is important in some animals as a means of conserving heat by the thermal insulation afforded by the trapped air near the skin. It may also have a defence function in animals such as the lion where the mane appears much larger when piloerection occurs. In man, body hair is largely vestigal and pilo-erection is manifested by 'goose-pimples' in the skin which may be a response to cold or emotion and by the prickling feeling at the back of the head caused by pilo-erection of the hair during times of severe fear or emotion. Sympathetic stimulation increases sweat secretion by the eccrine glands. There is no parasympathetic nerve supply to any of these skin structures.

The thyroid gland
Sympathetic postganglionic fibres travel to the gland from the middle and superior cervical ganglia and parasympathetic preganglionic fibres arise from the dorsal nucleus of the vagus in the medulla. The parasympathetic preganglionic fibres synapse with the cell bodies of postganglionic neurones which are diffusely situated in the gland and its vasculature. It appears that the majority of autonomic fibres, both sympathetic and parasympathetic, innervate the vasculature of the gland, the sym-

pathetic fibres causing vasoconstriction and the parasympathetic vasodilatation. However, there is some evidence that sympathetic fibres may have a minor role in the secretion of thyroid hormone.

Thoracic viscera

Heart

Sympathetic fibres emerge from the spinal cord with the upper five or six thoracic white rami, enter the paravertebral sympathetic chains and synapse with the three cervical ganglia and with the upper five or six thoracic ganglia. The heart therefore receives postganglionic sympathetic fibres from a wide area. The postganglionic sympathetic fibres end around the conducting tissues of the heart and also diffusely in the muscle fibres of both atria and ventricles. The parasympathetic supply to the heart is from the vagus, the preganglionic fibres of which synapse with the diffusely arranged ganglion cells situated on the atria. From these ganglion cells postganglionic fibres arise which innervate the conducting tissues of the heart; the pacemaker (*sino-atrial node*), the atrial-ventricular bundle (*Bundle of His*). There is little evidence in man of direct innervation of ventricular muscle by parasympathetic fibres.

Effects of autonomic stimulation. Sympathetic stimulation increases pacemaker activity and increases the rate of conduction of impulses through the conducting tissue leading to *tachycardia* (increased heart-rate). In addition, the force of contraction of cardiac muscle is increased resulting in increased cardiac output. In man the cardiac sympathetic nerves appear to innervate the corresponding sides of the heart. The sympathetic nerves on the right side are more important in increasing heart-rate than those on the left, whilst the left cardiac sympathetic nerves end mostly in ventricular muscle and stimulation of them causes increased systolic blood pressure due to increased cardiac output with little effect on heart rate.

Parasympathetic stimulation causes *bradycardia* (slowing of the heart rate) by virtue of its effect on the pacemaker, reduced contractility of the atria and slowing of the rate of conduction through the atria and Bundle of His. Parasympathetic stimulation therefore causes a reduction in cardiac output. Changes in heart rate produced by nerve stimulation or by drugs are known as *chronotropic* effects and changes in the force of myocardial contractility as *inotropic* effects. Stimulation and inhibition of each type of effect are referred to as positive or negative respectively. Thus, sympathetic stimulation produces both positive chronotropic and inotropic effects.

The coronary blood vessels
The coronary blood vessels which supply the cardiac muscle with blood receive both sympathetic and parasympathetic (vagal) postganglionic fibres. However, the effects of autonomic stimulation on the calibre of the coronary vessels is complicated by the changes in the contractile state of the heart produced by nerve stimulation which may secondarily affect coronary vessel calibre. In general, sympathetic stimulation produces dilatation of coronary vessels whilst parasympathetic stimulation produces constriction. However, most authorities are agreed that the local production of vasodilator metabolites as a result of increased myocardial contractility is the main mechanism whereby sympathetic stimulation produces coronary vasodilatation. The parasympathetic innervation of the coronary vessels is poorly developed and its function is not clear.

Respiratory system
Sympathetic preganglionic fibres arise from the upper four or five thoracic segments, traverse the corresponding white rami and synapse in the upper four or five thoracic ganglia and, to a lesser extent, in the cervical chain ganglia. Postganglionic fibres from these ganglia travel to the pulmonary plexuses around the hilus of the lung and finally end in the smooth muscle of the trachea, bronchi and bronchioles. Parasympathetic fibres from the vagus synapse in the anterior and posterior plexuses about the bronchi. Postganglionic parasympathetic fibres innervate the smooth muscle of the respiratory tract and also the mucus-secreting glands lining it.
Effects of autonomic stimulation. Sympathetic stimulation relaxes the smooth muscle of the respiratory tract causing bronchodilatation whilst parasympathetic stimulation causes bronchoconstriction and increased flow of mucus from the bronchial glands.

The limbs
The sympathetic supply to the arms arises from the upper thoracic region of the cord with segments three to six supplying most of the preganglionic fibres. The postganglionic sympathetic fibres arise from the middle and inferior cervical ganglia and

from the upper two, and sometimes three, thoracic ganglia. The sympathetic postganglionic fibres pass into the brachial plexus and innervate blood vessels in the muscle and skin, the sweat glands and pilomotor muscles.

The legs receive a sympathetic supply via the lower thoracic and upper lumbar segments of the cord. The connector fibres end in the lumbar and sacral ganglia of the sympathetic chain. The excitor fibres arise here and join the lumbosacral plexus, and are thus distributed to the leg, innervating the same structures as in the arm.

Effects of autonomic stimulation. The effects of sympathetic stimulation in the arms and legs is to cause vasoconstriction in the large arteries and in most of the vessels of the skin. However, some skin vessels and many vessels serving skeletal muscle are dilated by sympathetic stimulation. Sweat production is stimulated and piloerection occurs.

Gastrointestinal tract

Oesophagus
The connector cells of the sympathetic leave the cord mainly from the fourth to the sixth thoracic segments and synapse in the thoracic ganglia of the sympathetic chains and in the coeliac ganglion. Postganglionic fibres pass from the upper chain ganglia directly to the upper oesophagus. Other postganglionic sympathetic fibres reach the lower oesophagus mainly from the coeliac ganglion. Parasympathetic preganglionic fibres travel in the vagi and synapse with the diffusely arranged excitor cell bodies in the wall of the oesophagus. Postganglionic fibres arising from these ganglia pass to smooth muscle throughout the organ and to its cardiac sphincter.

Effects of autonomic stimulation. Sympathetic stimulation causes increased tone of the cardiac sphincter, diminishes tone and motility in the lower third of the organ and augments contraction produced by vagal contraction of the upper third. The sympathetic fibres to the lower part of the oesophagus appear to innervate mainly the blood vessels in this region and changes in tone produced by sympathetic stimulation may be, at least partly, secondary to changes in blood flow. Parasympathetic stimulation causes increased tone and motility of the upper and lower thirds of the organ and relaxation with an after effect of strong contraction in the cardiac sphincter.

Stomach and intestines

Sympathetic preganglionic fibres innervating the stomach, small intestine, ascending and transverse colon arise from the fifth or sixth to the tenth or eleventh thoracic segments. Most of these preganglionic fibres pass through the paravertebral sympathetic chains without synapsing and emerge as the splanchnic nerves which travel to the coeliac and mesenteric plexuses in the abdomen. Postganglionic fibres arising from these plexuses pass through the mesentery, usually accompanying blood vessels, to the smooth muscle of the intestinal tract. The descending colon, sigmoid, and rectum are supplied with preganglionic fibres from the first two and sometimes three lumbar segments of the cord. A few of these fibres synapse in the sympathetic chains but the majority pass through in the splanchnic nerves and synapse in the inferior mesenteric, hypogastric and pelvic plexuses.

Parasympathetic preganglionic fibres travel with the vagus through the coeliac and mesenteric plexuses to synapse with the intrinsic neurones in the myenteric (Auerbach's) plexus situated between the longitudinal and circular muscle coats of the gastrointestinal tract. The lower part of the intestinal tract, from the descending colon to the rectum, receive preganglionic parasympathetic fibres from the second to fourth sacral segments which pass via the pelvic nerves to the postganglionic neurones in the pelvic plexus and in Auerbach's plexus.

Effects of autonomic stimulation. Sympathetic nerve stimulation inhibits peristaltic movements and increases the tone of the sphincters. It does not inhibit gastric secretions but may have some inhibitory effect on the secretion of other digestive juices. Parasympathetic stimulation increases peristaltic activity and the secretion of gastric and other digestive juices but decreases the tone of the sphincters.

Peristaltic movements and movements involved in emptying the gut of waste materials are mainly initiated by local reflexes caused by distension of the gut lumen with either food or faeces. The afferent (sensory) neurones of the reflex are present in the submucous (Meissner's) plexus and these make synaptic connections with the cell bodies of the excitor neurones in Auerbach's plexus. This so-called *peristaltic reflex* can occur without any neural connections to the brain or spinal cord and was demonstrated by Trendelelburg (1917) in isolated segments of intestine. The extrinsic nerves to the gastrointestinal tract appear to have only a minor role in modulating activity of the organ.

The adrenal medullae
Sympathetic preganglionic fibres for the adrenal glands arise from the mid and lower thoracic segments and travel mainly with the lesser splanchnic nerve to traverse the coeliac and adrenal plexuses to reach the adrenal medullae. A small number of the preganglionic fibres synapse with scattered postganglionic neurones in the capsule of the gland and in the medulla. The postganglionic fibres from these cells innervate the blood vessels of the gland. The majority of preganglionic fibres end on the chromaffin cells of the medulla which serve the function of postganglionic neurones. The cortex of the adrenal gland is not directly innervated.

Effects of autonomic stimulation. Sympathetic preganglionic stimulation to the adrenal gland leads to the release of adrenaline and noradrenaline into the bloodstream from whence they circulate to smooth muscle containing structures in various parts of the body. The effects of these circulating hormones is, in many ways, to imitate and reinforce the effects of sympathetic stimulation. There is evidence to suggest that adrenaline and noradrenaline are stored in different types of chromaffin cells and that discrete areas of the hindbrain control the secretion of each.

The blood vessels of the splanchnic region
The sympathetic system contains many preganglionic fibres which synapse in the sympathetic chain and in the abdominal plexuses and which then innervate the blood vessels supplying the abdominal viscera. The arterioles in this region, because of their small calibre and large number, contribute a large proportion of the total vascular resistance (i.e. *peripheral resistance*) in the body and are therefore important in maintaining the level of systemic arterial blood pressure. The calibre of these vessels is controlled entirely by the sympathetic innervation which has a vasoconstrictor function.

Gall bladder and bile duct
Sympathetic preganglionic fibres arise from the lower thoracic segments and pass via the splanchnic nerves to synapse in the coeliac ganglion from whence postganglionic fibres pass to the gall bladder and ducts. Parasympathetic fibres from the vagus pass through the coeliac plexus and synapse in the intrinsic plexus in the walls of the bladder and its ducts. Sympathetic stimulation inhibits the musculature of the biliary tract whilst

parasympathetic stimulation increases the tone and motility of the gall bladder and inhibits contraction of the sphincter.

Liver and pancreas

The liver receives only a sympathetic nerve supply whilst the pancreas receives fibres from both sympathetic and parasympathetic systems. The sympathetic supply arises from thoracic segments five to nine (T5 to T9) and passes by way of the greater splanchnic nerve to synapse in the coeliac plexus. The postganglionic sympathetic fibres mostly innervate the blood vessels in the pancreas but in the liver many of the cells of the organ are directly innervated. The pancreas receives a parasympathetic supply from the vagus.

Effects of autonomic stimulation. Sympathetic stimulation of the liver causes an increase in blood glucose level due to an increased breakdown of glycogen. The increased breakdown of glycogen is thought to be due to sympathetic activation of the enzyme *adenyl cyclase.* In the presence of adenyl cyclase adenosinetriphosphate (*ATP*) is broken down to cyclic 3,5-adenosinemonophosphate (cyclic-3,5-AMP) which activates liver *phosphorylase* which in turn promotes the breakdown of glycogen. In the pancreas, sympathetic stimulation causes mainly vasoconstriction whilst parasympathetic stimulation promotes the secretion of pancreatic juices and insulin.

Adipose tissue

The fat stores in the omentum and at other sites receive a sympathetic innervation, the origin of which depends on the position of the fat. Sympathetic stimulation, by a mechanism similar to that producing glycolysis in the liver, leads to an increase in blood level of free fatty acids due to breakdown of fats by a lipase enzyme.

Spleen

The sympathetic postganglionic fibres to this organ arise from the coeliac ganglion and innervate the smooth muscle of the splenic capsule and the trabeculae. Sympathetic stimulation causes contraction of the splenic capsule resulting in the expulsion of erythrocytes stored in the splenic sinuses.

The kidneys

These organs receive a rich sympathetic supply which arises from spinal segments from the fourth thoracic segment to the second lumbar segments (T4 to L2) with most fibres originating from T10 to T12. The preganglionic fibres synapse in the coeliac ganglion, the superior and inferior mesenteric ganglia and in the renal plexus; postganglionic fibres innervate the vasculature of the kidneys. The precise role of the vasoconstrictor fibres to the renal vasculature is not certain and it is thought that autoregulatory mechanisms may have a more important effect on intra-renal blood flow. There is recent evidence which suggests that renal sympathetic nerve stimulation may induce release of the proteolytic enzyme *renin* from the juxtaglomerular cells of the kidney.

Urinary bladder
Sympathetic preganglionic fibres arise from the lower thoracic and upper two or three lumbar segments and for the most part pass through the sympathetic chains and synapse in the inferior mesenteric, hypogastric and vesical ganglia from all of which postganglionic fibres pass to the wall of the bladder. Para-sympathetic preganglionic fibres leave the spinal cord from the sacral outflow as the pelvic nerves which synapse with the cell bodies of postganglionic neurones in the wall of the bladder.

Effects of autonomic stimulation. The precise role of the autonomic nerves in the control of micturition is a subject of some debate. Sympathetic fibres innervate the vasculature of the bladder and also some areas of the bladder wall although in man at least, there is little evidence of sympathetic innervation of the detrusor muscle. Stimulation of the sympathetic nerves to the bladder causes the ureteral orifices to close and the base of the bladder to be pulled down. Parasympathetic stimulation causes a contraction of the detrusor muscle and a relaxation of the sphincter thus aiding emptying of the bladder. The external sphincters of the bladder and the perineal muscles are under conscious control so that micturation is a complex mechanism involving autonomic and somatic nervous systems.

Reproductive system
Sympathetic preganglionic fibres leave the spinal cord with the white rami of the lower thoracic and upper lumbar cord segments. Most of these fibres pass through the sympathetic chains without synapsing and terminate around the cell bodies of ganglion cells in the inferior mesenteric, hypogastric and preaortic plexuses and with scattered ganglion cells around the tissues innervated. From these various sites postganglionic fibres

arise and are distributed to the vasa deferentia, ejaculatory ducts, seminal vesicles, prostate gland and testes of the male and to the uterus, fallopian tubes, vestibular glands of the vagina and blood vessels of the clitoris, uterus and vagina in the female.

The parasympathetic supply is derived from the sacral outflow and passes via the pelvic nerves and nervi erigentes to the diffusely arranged pelvic plexuses. Postganglionic fibres innervate the blood vessels of the cavernous bodies of the penis in the male and the clitoris and possibly the wall of the uterus in the female.

Effects of autonomic stimulation. In the male sympathetic stimulation causes vasoconstriction and contraction of the smooth muscles of the prostate, seminal vesicles, prostatic urethra and vas deferens. The parasympathetic system promotes vasodilatation of the blood vessels of the cavernous tissue of the penis and thus promotes penile erection. Erection is maintained by passive compression of the veins from the cavernous tissue thus reducing venous outflow. The sympathetic system is therefore of most importance in effecting ejaculation and the parasympathetic in maintaining penile erection. Somatic nerves are also important in ejaculation since semen is ejected by the rhythmic contractions of the bulbo- and ischio-cavernous muscles which compress the urethra. The sympathetic system prevents passage of ejaculate into the bladder by increasing the tone of the bladder internal sphincter and also brings about subsidence of erection by increasing vasoconstriction in the arteries of the erectile tissue.

In the female sympathetic stimulation contracts the uterus and fallopian tubes and increases secretion of mucus from the vestibular glands. The parasympathetic innervation has a doubtful function in the uterus but is responsible for the erection of the clitoris which is the female equivalent of the penis. The significance of the autonomic innervation to the uterus is unclear since the organ is reported to function normally when all extrinsic nervous connections have been sectioned.

Homeostatic role of the autonomic nervous system

As mentioned previously in this chapter, Gaskell's concept of sympathetic and parasympathetic systems exerting opposing effects on smooth muscle and tending to cancel each others effects, is an over-simplification of the known facts. In practice the two systems work closely in concert with each other rather than opposition to produce a level of activity in the effector organ appropriate to maintain homeostasis. Autonomic influence on the heart rate is a good example of this co-operative working. On moderate exercise the tachycardia which occurs is mainly due to withdrawal of inhibitory vagal tone whereas with more severe exercise there is an additional increase in sympathetic activity. Both divisions of the autonomic system work closely together and also with the somatic system in producing the complex adjustments necessary for such functions as ejaculation, defaecation and micturation.

Cannon's vivid description of intense sympathetic activity as the fight or flight syndrome has served as a useful aid to memorise sympathetic effects but has similarly led to some misconceptions regarding the more usual role of the sympathetic system in the maintenance of homeostasis. Although capable of the dramatic effects described by Cannon, the sympathetic system is constantly effecting small undramatic effects such as the adjustment of blood flow to tissues. An analogy which has been used to describe sympathetic function likens it to man riding a bicycle who constantly makes small adjustments to maintain his balance but is also capable of very violent and sudden adjustments should he skid on a patch of oil.

Loss of autonomic function
Much has been written concerning the consequences of loss of autonomic function and the concensus of opinion suggests that partial autonomic loss is not fatal in most species but the ability to maintain homeostasis is greatly impaired and the animal is therefore less able to withstand adverse conditions such as lowering or raising of the ambient temperature. Cannon (1932) removed large portions of the sympathetic system from cats by removing the paravertebral ganglionic chains and found that they survived providing they were not unduly stressed. Many later studies have confirmed Cannon's observations regarding the effects of partial sympathectomy. Sympathectomy has been produced either surgically or, more recently, by the use of drugs such as 6-hydroxydopamine which has a specific effect in destroying sympathetic nerve terminals. A serum has also been developed containing a factor essential for the development of nerves which is able to stimulate the production of antibodies to it when injected into animals during the first few days of life. The effect of immunisation with anti nerve-growth factor is that the development of the sympathetic system, which usually occurs in the early days of life, is largely prevented. The homeo-

static consequences of this treatment largely confirms the results obtained using sympathectomy or 6-hydroxydopamine.

It is virtually impossible to produce a corresponding parasympathectomy by surgical techniques because of the diffuse and widespread distribution of the parasympathetic ganglion cells. Possibly the closest approximation to complete loss of the autonomic nervous system may be achieved by drugs such as hexamethonium, which prevent the passage of impulses across all autonomic ganglia (Chapter 7). These drugs were formerly much used to treat high blood pressure (*hypertension*) in man. In clinical use they produced a formidable range of unwanted effects due to loss of autonomic function and, in full dosage, sometimes produced a fatal paralysis of the intestine.

SUMMARY

The peripheral sympathetic nerves in man arise from the 12 thoracic and upper 3 lumbar segments of the vertebral column (*thoracico-lumbar sympathetic outflow*). In general, the preganglionic sympathetic fibres from the cord synapse either with one or more sympathetic ganglia in the paravertebral sympathetic chains or with prevertebral ganglia, such as the coeliac and mesenteric ganglia in the abdominal cavity.

The peripheral parasympathetic nerves arise from the brain (in cranial nerves III, VII, IX and X) and from the second to fourth sacral cord segments (*cranio-sacral parasympathetic outflow*). The vagi (cranial nerve X) are the most important and widespread parasympathetic nerves and innervate many tissues including the heart, stomach and much of the intestine. The sympathetic system is mainly concerned with functions involving increased activity of tissues used in states of high bodily activity such as stimulation of the force and rate of the heart during exercise. The parasympathetic system is mainly concerned with more sedentary activities such as digestion and emptying of bladder and bowel. Many tissues receive fibres from each division of the autonomic nervous system having opposing effects when stimulated; the heart, pupil and intestine are examples. Other tissues are innervated predominantly by one or other division, e.g. most blood vessels receive only a sympathetic (vasoconstrictor) innervation. In still other organs, such as the uterus, the autonomic innervation has an obscure and apparently minor role to play in the activity of the tissue.

Experimental evidence using both drugs and surgical procedures suggests that the autonomic nervous system, although probably not essential for life, plays an important role in the maintenance of homeostasis. It is evident that the parasympathetic and sympathetic divisions of the autonomic nervous system work in concert, rather than in opposition, to produce changes in bodily function.

REFERENCES

Cannon, W. B. (1929) Organization for physiological homeostasis. *Physiol. Rev.*, **9**, 399–431.
Cannon, W. B. (1932) *The Wisdom of the Body.* London: Kegan Paul, Trench, Trubner & Co. Ltd.
Gaskell, W. H. (1886) On the structure, distribution and function of the nerves which innervate the visceral and vascular systems. *J. Physiol.*, **7**, 1–80.
Meyer, H. H. & Gottlieb, R. (1911) *Die Experimentelle Pharmakologie.* 2. Aufl. Berlin: Urban & Schwarzenberg.
Trendelenburg, P. (1917) Physiologische und pharmakologische versuche über die dünndarmperistaltik. *Arch. Expt. Pathol. Pharmakol.*, **81**, 55–129.

GENERAL READING

Cannon, W. B. (1929) *Bodily Changes in Pain, Hunger, Fear and Rage.* 2nd edn., New York: D. Appleton and Company.
Kuntz, A. (1953) *The Autonomic Nervous System.* 4th edn., Philadelphia: Lee & Febiger.
Mitchell, G. A. G. (1953) *Anatomy of the Autonomic Nervous System.* Edinburgh: E. & S. Livingstone Ltd.
Peele, L. T. (1961) *The Neuroanatomic Basis for Clinical Neurology.* 2nd edn., Chapter 7, pp 146–170. New York: McGraw-Hill Book Co. Inc.
Truex, R. C. & Carpenter, M. B. (1969) *Human Neuroanatomy.* 6th edn., Chapter 11, pp 216–235. Baltimore: The Williams & Wilkins Company.

3

Neurohumoral transmission in the autonomic nervous system

'Of known natural processes that might pass on excitation, only two are, in my opinion, worth talking about: either there exists at the boundary of the contractile substance a stimulatory secretion in the form of a thin layer of ammonia, lactic acid, or some other powerful stimulatory substance; or the phenomenon is electrical in nature.'

This prophetic statement was made by E. Du Bois-Reymond in 1877 and it clearly outlines the stage of knowledge concerning the neurotransmission process at that time and also states the two most likely explanations of the problem which were to occupy many physiologists for the following 70 years or so. At the time that Du Bois-Reymond made this statement it was already known, from the work of Claude Bernard and others, that electrical stimulation of nerves could influence the activity of both smooth and striated (skeletal) muscle. What was not clear, however, was how electrical activity produced in nerves could be transmitted to muscles.

It can now be stated with some confidence that as regards higher mammalian species, including man, transmission of impulses from nerve to nerve and from nerve to muscle is effected by the release from nerve endings of highly active substances called *neurotransmitters*. However, the road to acceptance of the 'chemical' rather than the 'electrical' theory of neurotransmission has been a long and difficult one.

HISTORICAL OUTLINE OF THE DEVELOPMENT OF THE NEUROHUMORAL THEORY OF TRANSMISSION

The inner part (medulla) of the mammalian adrenal gland contains considerable amounts of the sympathetic neurotransmitter substance noradrenaline as well as much larger amounts of the chemically-related adrenaline. Thus it is not surprising that the first experimental evidence concerning the theory of neurohumoral transmission should come from experiments using extracts of adrenal glands nor indeed that the wrong substance (adrenaline) should be initially chosen as the most likely candidate. Oliver & Schäfer (1895) first reported on the physiological effects of injecting extracts of adrenal glands into cats and Lewandowsky (1898) extended these observations by noting the similarity of the effects produced by these extracts with the effects produced by stimulating sympathetic nerves. Langley (1901) confirmed these observations and suggested that the extracts might be acting by stimulating sympathetic nerve endings. In the same year Takamine (1901) isolated, in relatively pure form, the active principle of the adrenal extract which he called *adrenalin*. In 1904 T. R. Elliott, at that time a young Research Fellow working in Langley's Department at Cambridge, made two classical observations concerning the effects of adrenaline. Firstly, he showed that it had little effect on smooth muscle which was not sympathetically-innervated, and secondly, that adrenaline retained its activity when tested on tissues normally receiving sympathetic fibres but in which the post-ganglionic sympathetic nerves had previously been sectioned and allowed to degenerate. This latter observation was inconsistent with Langley's previous suggestion of adrenaline acting by stimulating sympathetic nerve endings. Elliott suggested that adrenaline might be the chemical stimulant released when electrical impulses reach the end of sympathetic nerves. Obviously, Langley and Elliott mutually influenced each others thinking on the subject. In his Croonian lecture to the Royal Society in 1906 Langley made it clear that he considered the release of chemical substances from nerve endings to be a possible explanation of the nerve-muscle transmission process. Moreover, in the same lecture he propounded the theory of specific areas on muscles at which drugs might act to initiate effects on muscle activity. These areas he called 'receptive substances' from which arises the modern concept of drug receptors.

At about the same time similar inconclusive observations suggesting the release of a chemical substance from parasympathetic nerve endings were being reported. Schmeideberg & Koppe (1869) reported on the similarity between the effects after injection into animals of the substance *muscarine*, obtained from the fungus Amanita muscaria, and the effects produced by electrical stimulation of the vagus and of their common antagonism by atropine. W. E. Dixon (1907) was almost certainly aware of these experiments and of Elliott's concept of neuro-humoral transmission. Accordingly, he attempted to demonstrate the release of amuscarine-like substance from the cardiac vagus after electrical stimulation. Animals (species not stated) were killed by pithing, bled and the cardiac vagus stimulated for half an hour. The heart was then removed, briefly immersed in boiling water and extracted with ethanol. After removal of the ethanol the residue was dissolved in saline and was found to cause slowing of an isolated frog heart. The inhibitory effect of the extract was abolished by atropine and disappeared if the solution were left standing in the laboratory for 24 hours. Unfortunately, Dixon's very brief account gives insufficient details of his methodology to decide whether or not he had made the first demonstration of neurohumoral transmission. It is curious that Dixon did not persist with this very promising line of investigation or publish a fuller account of his experimental results.

Thus the conceptual ground had been prepared for the demonstration of the phenomenon of neurohumoral transmission but convincing experimental evidence was still lacking. This evidence was finally provided in 1921 by the elegantly simple and direct experiments of the German physiologist Otto Loewi. According to Loewi, the idea for the experiment came to him in the middle of the night. He took the isolated hearts from two frogs; these were cannulated and filled with Ringer's solution and then set up to allow of the mechanical recording of their rate and amplitude of beating. In one heart Loewi prepared the vago-sympathetic trunk for electrical stimulation. This nerve contains both sympathetic and parasympathetic fibres but when stimulated it was the parasympathetic effect which predominated and the force and rate of the heart-beat were reduced. After stimulation of the first heart in this way, Loewi pipetted some of the Ringer solution from this heart and transferred it to the cannula of the second heart and found that this heart was also inhibited. Loewi suggested that the inhibition of the second heart was brought about by release of a chemical substance, which he called '*vagusstoff*', into the perfusate of the stimulated heart. In later experiments, using frogs at a different season of the year, Loewi showed that the predominant effect of vago-sympathetic stimulation was increased cardiac force and rate and this effect, too, could be transferred in the perfusate from a stimulated to a non-stimulated heart. The cardiac excitatory substance Loewi called '*acceleranstoff*' and later he suggested that it might be adrenaline.

Loewi's experiments took some time to gain universal acceptance as proof of neurohumoral transmission. The records of his experiments were not entirely convincing and the crude methodology combined with the seasonal variations in frogs made his experiments open to criticism and difficult to confirm. However, confirmation and gradual acceptance of the theory came over the next 10 years or so. Bacq (1975) has traced in detail the development of the theory of neurohumoral transmission and has pointed out that in the choice of species and experimental conditions Loewi was fortunate. Frog heart contains only a small amount of the enzyme cholinesterase and the low temperature used reduces its activity in hydrolysing acetylcholine released from the parasympathetic nerve endings. Moreover, the use of Ringer solution, in place of blood, for the perfusate removed a rich source of cholinesterase from the experiment.

Identification of the neurotransmitter role of acetylcholine both in autonomic and somatic nerves was greatly aided by the discovery by Loewi & Navratil (1926) of the inhibitory action of eserine (also called physostigmine) on cholinesterase. The workers most prominent in these experiments were the German physiologists W. Feldberg and O. Krayer and the great English physiologist H. H. Dale. Dale's major contribution to our understanding of the physiology and pharmacology of autonomic transmitters came in 1914 when he clearly showed that acetylcholine produced two quite separate types of action in the body. In normal doses acetylcholine lowered the blood pressure of anaesthetised cats and this response, like that to muscarine, was readily abolished by atropine. However, after atropine, larger doses of acetylcholine raised the blood pressure and stimulated the heart and skeletal muscles. These effects resembled the effects of the alkaloid nicotine, were not blocked by atropine but were abolished after a large dose of nicotine. Thus acetylcholine had two sets of actions 'muscarine' actions and 'nicotine' actions. Later work by Dale and by others demonstrated that acetylcholine released from postganglionic parasympathetic nerve endings produced muscarinic effects susceptible to the blocking action of atropine, whilst acetylcholine released from preganglionic nerve endings in both sympathetic and parasympathetic systems produced nicotinic effects. Dale (1914) showed that part of the pressor response produced by large doses of acetylcholine after atropine was due to release of adrenaline from the cells of the adrenal medullae. The cells of the adrenal medullae which store adrenaline (and noradrenaline) behave like autonomic ganglion cells in as much as they are stimulated by acetylcholine released from preganglionic (splanchnic) nerve endings and acting upon nicotinic receptors. Transmission of impulses between somatic nerves and voluntary muscle is also mediated by acetylcholine having a nicotinic action.

Despite the rapidly growing body of evidence in favour of the concept of neurohumoral transmission which accumulated after the work of Loewi some eminent physiologists for many years maintained a steadfast preference for an electrical explanation of the phenomenon. Most notable amongst them was the Nobel laureate J. C. Eccles who did not concede conversion to the theory until 1945.

Identification of noradrenaline as the sympathetic postganglionic transmitter substance in mammals
Part of the opposition to the concept of neurohumoral transmission arose from discrepancies, in some tissues, between the effects produced by stimulating sympathetic nerves and those produced by adrenaline, the proposed transmitter substance. As early as 1910 Barger & Dale had examined the effects of a number of substances related to adrenaline and reported that one of them (noradrenaline) more faithfully reproduced the effects of sympathetic nerve stimulation than did adrenaline. Since noradrenaline was not at the time known to occur naturally in the body Dale wrongly interpreted this observation as evidence against the concept of neurohumoral transmission because it was inconsistent with Elliott's earlier suggestion of adrenaline as the transmitter substance released from postganglionic sympathetic nerve endings. Similar difficulties were encountered after the publication of Loewi's results and it was not until more refined chemical techniques were developed that von Euler (1946) was able to show that in higher mammals, including man, noradrenaline is the neurotransmitter released from sympathetic nerve endings. Ironically, modern chemical techniques have proved Loewi to be right in as much that in the frog, as in certain other lower species, the sympathetic neurotransmitter is in fact adrenaline.

Terminology
Dale (1933) suggested the terms '*cholinergic*' to describe nerves releasing acetylcholine and '*adrenergic*' for those releasing adrenaline or a closely related substance. The word adrenergic has led to some confusion since its use was well established by the time

noradrenaline was positively identified as the postganglionic sympathetic transmitter. In this monograph the word *noradrenergic* will be used to describe nerves in which noradrenaline is known to be the transmitter. This distinction, largely academic until recently, may be of greater importance in the future since recent work suggests the presence of true adrenergic, i.e. adrenaline-releasing neurones in the brains of some mammalian species.

The concept of receptors

When neurotransmitters are released from nerves they are thought to combine with specialised sites on the postsynaptic cells to initiate the train of events producing the effects typical of stimulation of that type of nerve to that particular tissue. These specialised sites, called 'receptive areas' or 'receptive substances' by Langley, are now referred to simply as *receptors*. Substances other than neurotransmitters may activate receptors or may block them by occupying then without activation and thus prevent the access of activating substances such as drugs or neurotransmitters. Substances (i.e. drugs) which activate (stimulate) receptors are termed *agonists* and those which occupy receptors and block the effects of agonists are termed *antagonists*. Agonists may initiate either increased or decreased activity of a tissue depending on the type of receptor stimulated. Many drugs possess both agonist and antagonist activities. For example, nicotine was used by Langley in low doses to stimulate autonomic ganglia and in higher doses to block its own effects and to prevent transmission of impulses through autonomic ganglia. It has become increasingly obvious over the years that not all (possibly not even most) receptors are associated with nerve endings. Many receptors appear to be widely distributed throughout tissues and may be stimulated by substances, either naturally-occurring or otherwise, not yet identified as neurotransmitters. In general, receptors are classified according to the specificity of one type (or a group) of agonists and antagonists in stimulating and blocking them respectively.

Little is known about the physico-chemical nature, or indeed about the precise physiological functioning, of receptors. However, they have been of great conceptual importance to physiologists and pharmacologists in explaining and classifying the various actions of neurotransmitters. The receptor concept has also been of great value to pharmacologists and organic chemists in the design of many new drugs, both agonists and antagonists, some of which have been of great clinical importance.

Neurotransmitters in the mammalian autonomic nervous system

The neurotransmitters which have thus far been positively identified in the peripheral autonomic nervous system are acetylcholine and noradrenaline. The cells of the adrenal medullae release a mixture of adrenaline and noradrenaline into

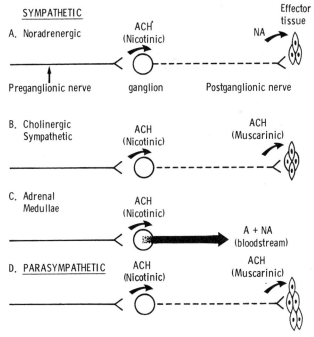

Fig. 3. 1 Neurotransmitters in the autonomic nervous system.
A, sympathetic preganglionic nerves release acetylcholine (ACH) which acts upon nicotinic receptors in the ganglia. The majority of postganglionic sympathetic nerves release noradrenaline (NA) at the neuro-effector junction (noradrenergic nerves).
B, a small number of postganglionic sympathetic nerves release acetylcholine acting upon muscarinic receptors at the neuro-effector junction (cholinergic sympathetic nerves).
C, the chromaffin cells of the adrenal medullae are innervated by preganglionic sympathetic fibres releasing acetylcholine and acting upon nicotinic receptors. The chromaffin cells release a mixture of adrenaline (A) and noradrenaline (NA) into the bloodstream.
D, in the parasympathetic system acetylcholine is the neurotransmitter both at the ganglionic synapse (nicotinic action) and at the neuro-effector junction (muscarinic action). Preganglionic nerves are indicated by solid lines and postganglionic by broken lines.

the bloodstream but since, in this case, they are widely distributed in the body they are usually thought of as hormones in this context rather than as neurotransmitters.

The sites of release of acetylcholine and noradrenaline in the autonomic nervous system are shown in Fig. 3.1. Acetylcholine is released from preganglionic nerve endings of both sympathetic and parasympathetic systems and from the preganglionic nerves innervating the cells of the adrenal medullae. All these effects of acetylcholine are mimicked by *nicotine*, the alkaloid from the tobacco plant, and are termed *nicotinic actions* of acetylcholine. The receptors on the postsynaptic cells on which this acetylcholine acts are called *nicotinic receptors*. The nicotinic actions of acetylcholine are abolished by large doses of nicotine itself or by ganglion blocking drugs such as *hexamethonium*, but are unaffected by atropine.

Postganglionic parasympathetic nerves also release acetylcholine as their neurotransmitter substance and these effects are mimicked by the fungal alkaloid *muscarine*. These effects of acetylcholine are therefore called *muscarinic actions* and the receptors acted upon, *muscarinic receptors*. The muscarinic actions of acetylcholine are abolished by atropine but are unaffected by hexamethonium. Some autonomic nerves, anatomically sympathetic, release acetylcholine instead of noradrenaline as their transmitter substance. These cholinergic sympathetic nerves innervate the sweat glands of the skin and also some blood vessels and the acetylcholine they release acts upon muscarinic receptors, hence the inhibition of sweat secretion after atropine.

The majority of sympathetic nerves are *noradrenergic*, i.e. they release noradrenaline as their neurotransmitter substance from postganglionic fibres.

Neurohumoral transmission in somatic nerves supplying skeletal muscle

Acetylcholine is the neurotransmitter substance released from somatic nerves supplying skeletal (voluntary) muscle. The effects of acetylcholine released from these nerves are mediated via stimulation of receptors, classified by Langley as nicotinic. However, the effects of stimulating nicotinic receptors in skeletal muscle are more readily abolished by *curare*, a plant extract, than by ganglion blocking drugs such as hexamethonium. Curare is termed a neuromuscular blocking drug and d-tubocurarine the active constituent isolated from it finds clinical use to produce muscular relaxation during surgery. Curare possesses autonomic ganglion blocking activity in doses only moderately higher than those needed to cause muscular relaxation and, conversely, hexamethonium which was formerly used clinically to block transmission through autonomic ganglia, in very high doses produced weakness of skeletal muscles in some patients. Thus, despite the fact that nicotine stimulates the acetylcholine receptors in both autonomic ganglia and in skeletal muscle, the differences in relative sensitivity to blockade by drugs such as d-tubocurarine and hexamethonium suggest that the two types of receptor are not identical.

The Burn-Rand hypothesis of cholinergic sympathetic transmission

As mentioned earlier a small number of nerves, anatomically sympathetic, such as those to the sweat glands of the skin have been shown to release acetylcholine instead of noradrenaline from their postganglionic endings. It was von Euler & Gaddum (1931) who first conclusively demonstrated the existence of these nerves. They showed that vasodilatation could be produced in the lips and buccal mucous membrane of the anaesthetised dog by stimulation of the superior cervical nerve and that this effect was due to acetylcholine release. Many other workers, both before and since 1931, using a variety of experimental tissues and conditions, reported acetylcholine-like responses on stimul- ation of sympathetic nerves and it seems likely that many, if not all, sympathetic nerves contain cholinergic fibres. These ob- servations have been extensively re-examined and extended in the years since 1959 largely as a result of the studies of J. H. Burn and M. J. Rand. These two pharmacologists, based on evidence from their conjoint work and that in association with a number of other workers, have propounded the hypothesis (known as the Burn-Rand or cholinergic-link hypothesis) that all sympathetic nerves release acetylcholine, which in most of them further initiates the release of noradrenaline.

The evidence in favour of the hypothesis has been largely gained from pharmacological studies and has been elegantly and persuasively reviewed by Burn (1975). The major evidence favouring the mediation of acetylcholine in noradrenaline re- lease from sympathetic nerves may be briefly summarised as follows:

1. In a variety of smooth muscle preparations, in both *in vitro* and *in vivo* studies, when the usual effects of sympathetic stimulation to a tissue are abolished by drugs such as guane-

thidine, which prevents transmitter release, or by reserpine, which depletes neuronal noradrenaline stores, then the effects of sympathetic stimulation often change to resemble those to cholinergic nerve stimulation. This is illustrated in Fig. 3.2 in which the sympathetic nerves to a loop of rabbit isolated intestine have been stimulated, resulting initially in cessation of the spontaneous (myogenic) contractions of the smooth muscle.

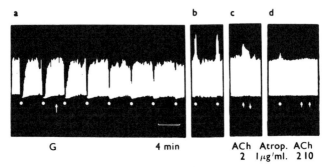

Fig. 3.2 Acetylcholine-like responses obtained from stimulating sympathetic noradrenergic nerves. The records are of the spontaneous contractions of the longitudinal muscle of a segment of rabbit isolated ileum suspended in Kreb's solution. At the white dots the sympathetic postganglionic nerves to the tissue were electrically stimulated for 14 seconds which initially inhibited the contractions. At G, guanethidine, a drug which prevents noradrenaline release from sympathetic nerves, was added to the solution bathing the tissue and the inhibitory responses to sympathetic stimulation were gradually abolished and eventually replaced by stimulant responses (in b). The stimulant effects of sympathetic stimulation, like those to added acetylcholine, were abolished by atropine, an antagonist of muscarinic acetylcholine receptors (panels c and d). (Taken from Day & Rand, 1961).

Guanethidine, a noradrenergic neurone blocking drug (see Chapter 10) abolished these typical effects of sympathetic stimulation and they were replaced by increase in the height of the muscle contractions during the periods of stimulation. These stimulant effects were probably due to activation of cholinergic fibres, present in the sympathetic nerves and revealed by guanethidine. The motor effects of sympathetic stimulation and the responses to added acetylcholine were both abolished by atropine, a muscarinic receptor blocking drug.

2. Acetylcholine and the enzyme acetylcholinesterase which normally destroys it in the body have both been detected in extracts of some sympathetic nerves. In addition, there have been several claims that acetylcholine itself has been detected in blood draining from organs after their sympathetic nerves have been stimulated.

3. Drugs such as hemicholinium, which interferes with acetylcholine synthesis, and botulinum toxin, which reduces acetylcholine release from cholinergic nerves, have been shown to reduce the responses to sympathetic nerve stimulation in some tissues. Similarly, it is known that calcium ions are necessary for acetylcholine release from cholinergic nerves and Burn and his colleagues have provided evidence that they are also necessary for normal functioning in noradrenergic nerves.

Burn (1975) considers that the cholinergic-link hypothesis is consistent with available evidence regarding the evolutionary development of the sympathetic noradrenergic system. It has been shown that in some lower species such as fish the sympathetic nerves to the gut are cholinergic whilst in some birds they may release both acetylcholine and a noradrenaline-like substance.

Many organisms during embryonic development or early in independent life are thought to go through developmental stages which trace evolutionary history of their species—'ontogeny recapitulates phylogeny'. In this respect it is interesting to note that in higher mammals, such as rabbits, the sympathetic nerves at birth contain little noradrenaline and when the supply to tissues such as the gut is stimulated the responses elicited closely resemble the responses to acetylcholine. Within a few weeks of birth the sympathetic nerves are able to synthesise and store noradrenaline and stimulation at this time evokes effects similar to those obtained in adult animals and closely resembling the responses obtained with noradrenaline.

Despite the attractive nature of the Burn-Rand hypothesis the weight of scientific opinion appears to be against its acceptance. The major criticisms of the hypothesis are firstly, that much of the pharmacological evidence could be accounted for by an admixture of noradrenergic and cholinergic fibres. The cholinergic fibres present in many sympathetic nerves could be of parasympathetic origin or be postganglionic cholinergic sympathetic fibres perhaps identical to those of the sweat glands. Secondly, much of the evidence in favour of the hypothesis is indirect in nature and has been obtained in tissues treated with substances such as hemicholinium and botulinum toxin and therefore relies heavily on the specificity of these pharmacological tools. For the hypothesis to gain more widespread support it would be necessary to conclusively demonstrate the presence of both acetylcholine and noradrenaline within the same sympathetic nerve fibre. This evidence is thus far lacking. However, whether the hypothesis can finally be substantiated or not, it has undoubtedly been very valuable in stimulating many important studies into the detailed functioning and anatomy of the autonomic nervous system.

Substances recently suggested to be neurotransmitters in the autonomic nervous system

In addition to the classical neurotransmitter substances acetylcholine and noradrenaline a number of other substances are now suspected of being neurotransmitters within the peripheral autonomic nervous system. Eccles (1964) has argued that any new candidate for the role of neurotransmitter must be able to satisfy a number of criteria:

1. The 'transmitter' and enzymes capable of its synthesis must be present in the nerve.
2. The 'transmitter' must be released when the nerves are stimulated.
3. The 'transmitter' given extrinsically must mimic the effect of nerve stimulation.
4. An enzyme or enzyme system capable of inactivating the proposed transmitter must be present in the tissue.
5. Drugs which alter the response to nerve stimulation should alter the response to the proposed transmitter in the same way.

Dopamine

Numerous studies in recent years have established that dopamine has important neurotransmitter functions in the brain as well as serving as the immediate synthetic precursor to noradrenaline in both brain and peripheral tissues. Bell & Lang (1973) made the first report concerning the possible existence of dopaminergic nerves outside of the central nervous system. These workers electrically stimulated the mid-brain area of anaesthetized dogs and found that it produced vasodilatation of the blood vessels supplying the kidneys, an effect apparently mediated by dopamine release from some of the renal nerves. Thorner (1975) has recently reviewed the evidence in favour of dopamine having an important function as a neurotransmitter substance in the autonomic nervous system.

5-Hydroxytryptamine (5-HT)

This substance, like dopamine, is generally accepted as having neurotransmitter functions within the brain. There is additional evidence, as yet inconclusive, that it may also act as a neurotransmitter in some autonomic ganglia and possibly also in autonomic nerves concerned with peristaltic movements of the intestine. If 5-HT gains general acceptance as a peripheral neurotransmitter substance then it is likely that the nerves releasing it will be termed 'tryptaminergic' as they already are for those present in the central nervous system.

Adenine nucleotides

In 1898 Langley demonstrated that the parasympathetic (vagal) nerves supplying the stomach of the cat contained inhibitory as well as motor fibres. This observation has since been confirmed in many other preparations of smooth muscle, mainly taken from the gastrointestinal tract. However, it was not until the advent, in the 1950's and 1960's, of drugs such as guanethidine and reserpine, which have relatively selective actions on noradrenergic nerves, that it became obvious that these effects were not due to the inclusion of noradrenergic fibres in the nerves stimulated. Burnstock and his colleagues have studied these nerves extensively and have concluded that they form part of the parasympathetic division of the autonomic nervous system and that the neurotransmitter substance released is adenosine triphosphate (ATP) or a closely related adenine nucleotide. Burnstock (1972) in a comprehensive review of the subject has suggested the name 'purinergic' to describe these nerves since the proposed neurotransmitter is a derivative of purine. The existence of 'purinergic' nerves is not yet established beyond doubt. Much of the experimental evidence in favour of the existence of these nerves has been derived from isolated smooth muscle tissues in which the nervous elements present have been stimulated by electrical currents passed throughout the tissue. It is likely that under these conditions many substances, possibly including those without neurotransmitter function, will be released and produce electrophysiological and activity changes in the smooth muscle. Another possibility which, as yet, has received little attention is that 'purinergic' responses might be mediated by substances released from sensory (afferent) nerves by impulses passing down them in the opposite direction to that normally travelled (i.e. antidromically). In this respect it is interesting to note that antidromic stimulation of the sensory nerves to the rabbit ear was shown by Holton (1959) to cause vasodilatation of the ear vessels and this effect was produced by the release of ATP from the nerves.

Certainly the existence of autonomic neurones releasing

adenine nucleotides is a fascinating possibility but they have not yet been demonstrated unequivocally and the use of the word 'purinergic' to describe them is probably premature.

Prostaglandins

These substances are widely distributed in the body and have been the subject of intense investigation over the past decade or so. They are derived from essential fatty acids such as arachidonic acid and at least a dozen different prostaglandins have been identified. They have widespread pharmacological effects in the body some of which may be of physiological consequence. It has been shown that they are released into the bloodstream when nerves, both somatic and autonomic, are stimulated. However, they are not themselves neurotransmitters since they are apparently released from the tissues and not from the nerve terminals. Prostaglandin E_2 is known to be released from the spleen when the sympathetic nerves are stimulated and Hedqvist (1970) showed that it inhibited noradrenaline release from the sympathetic nerve terminals and was probably responsible for the diminution in contractile responses of the spleen which occurred on repeated stimulation. The physiological significance, if any, of this and many similar observations will undoubtedly occupy many pharmacological 'man-hours' in the years ahead. Horton, whose group have contributed much to prostaglandin research, has reviewed (Horton, 1973) the effects of prostaglandins at sympathetic nerve endings.

SUMMARY

Impulse flow along autonomic nerve fibres is electrical in nature but transmission across synapses is effected by specific chemical substances (neurotransmitters) released by presynaptic nerve terminals. In the peripheral autonomic nervous system two substances, acetylcholine and noradrenaline, are known to act as neurotransmitters and recent research suggests that further substances will be positively identified in the future.

Acetylcholine is the neurotransmitter released from autonomic preganglionic nerves of both sympathetic and parasympathetic systems, including the preganglionic fibres which innervate the secretory cells of the adrenal medullae. At all these sites the actions of acetylcholine are mimicked by low doses of the alkaloid nicotine, are called nicotinic actions and act upon specialised structures on the postsynaptic cells called nicotinic receptors.

Nicotinic actions of acetylcholine within the autonomic nervous system are abolished by high concentrations of nicotine and by the drug hexamethonium.

Acetylcholine is also the neurotransmitter released from postganglionic parasympathetic nerves and from a minority of sympathetic nerves such as those to the sweat glands of the skin. These actions of acetylcholine are mimicked by the alkaloid muscarine and are therefore called muscarinic effects and the receptors acted upon muscarinic receptors. Muscarinic receptors are specifically blocked by the drug atropine. All nerves releasing acetylcholine, whether in the brain, somatic or autonomic systems, are referred to as cholinergic nerves.

Noradrenaline is the neurotransmitter released from most postganglionic sympathetic nerves and these nerves are now referred to as noradrenergic nerves in preference to the older and less precise term—adrenergic.

The adrenal medullae when stimulated release into the bloodstream predominantly adrenaline with a smaller amount of noradrenaline and these substances are able to produce widespread effects in the body which resemble and reinforce the effects produced by sympathetic nerve stimulation.

REFERENCES

Bacq, Z. M. (1975) *Chemical Transmission of Nerve Impulses.*, Oxford: Pergamon Press.

Barger, G. & Dale, H. H. (1910) Chemical structure and sympathomimetic action of amines. *J. Physiol.*, **41**, 19–59.

Bell, C. & Lang, W. J. (1973) Neural dopaminergic vasodilator control in the kidney. *Nature New Biology*, **246**, 27–29.

Burn, J. H. (1975) *The Autonomic Nervous System*, 5th edn., Oxford: Blackwell Scientific Publications.

Burnstock, G. (1972) Purinergic nerves, *Pharmac. Revs.*, **24**, 509–581.

Dale, H. H. (1914) The action of certain esters and ethers of choline, and their relation to muscarine. *J. Pharmac. exp. Ther.*, **2**, 147–190.

Dale, H. H. (1933) Nomenclature of fibres in the autonomic system and their effects. *J. Physiol.*, **80**, 10–11.

Day, M. D. & Rand, M. J. (1961) Effect of guanethidine in revealing cholinergic sympathetic fibres. *Br. J. Pharmac.*, **17**, 245–260.

Dixon, W. E. (1907) On the mode of action of drugs. *Medical Magazine (London)*, **16**, 454–457.

Du Bois-Reymond, E. (1877) *Gesammelte Abhandlungen der allgemeinen Muskel-und Nervenphysik*, **2**, 700.

Eccles, J. C. (1964) *The Physiology of Synapses*, Berlin: Springer-Verlag.

Elliott, T. R. (1904) The action of adrenalin. *J. Physiol.*, **32**, 401–467.

von Euler, U. S. (1946) A specific sympathomimetic ergone in adrenergic nerve fibres (sympathin) and its relations to adrenaline and noradrenaline. *Acta physiol. scand.*, **12**, 73–97.

von Euler, U. S. & Gaddum, J. H. (1931) Pseudomotor contractures after degeneration of the facial nerve. *J. Physiol.*, **73**, 54–66.

Hedqvist, P. (1970) Control by prostaglandin E_2 of sympathetic neurotransmission in the spleen. *Life Sciences*, **9**, part 1, 269–278.

Holton, Pamela (1959) The liberation of adenosine triphosphate on antidromic stimulation of sensory nerves. *J. Physiol.*, **145**, 494–504.

Horton, E. W. (1973) Prostaglandins at adrenergic nerve-endings. *Br. med. Bull.*, **29**, 148–151.

Langley, J. N. (1898) On inhibitory fibres in the vagus to the end of the oesophagus and stomach. *J. Physiol.*, **23**, 407–414.

Langley, J. N. (1901) Observations on the physiological action of extracts of the supra-renal bodies. *J. Physiol.*, **27**, 237–256.

Langley, J. N. (1906) Croonian lecture, on nerve endings and on special excitable substances in cells. *Proc. R. Soc. B.*, **78**, 170–194.

Lewandowsky, M. (1898) Ueber eine wirkung des nebennierenextractes auf das ange. *Zent Bl. Physiol.*, **12**, 599–600.

Loewi, O. (1921) Uebertragbarkeit der herznervenwirkung. *pflüg. Arch. ges. Physiol.*, **189**, 238–242.

Loewi, O. & Navratil, E. (1926) Uber humorale übertrag barkeit der herznervenwirkung. X. Uber das schicksal des vagusstoffes. *Pflüg. Arch. ges. Physiol.*, **214**, 678–688.

Oliver, G. & Schäfer, E. A. (1895) The physiological effects of extracts from the suprarenal capsules. *J. Physiol.*, **18**, 230–276.

Schmiedeberg, O. & Koppe, R. (1869) Das muscarin, das giftige alkaloid des fliegenpilzes. Leipzig: F. C. W. Vogel.

Takamine, J. (1901) The isolation of the active principle of the suprarenal gland. *J. Physiol.*, **27**, 29–30P.

Thorner, M. O. (1975) Dopamine is an important neurotransmitter in the autonomic nervous system. *Lancet*, **1**, 662–665.

GENERAL READING

Bacq, Z. M. (1975) *Chemical Transmission of Nerve Impulses*. Oxford: Pergamon Press.

Burn, J. H. (1975) *The Autonomic Nervous System*, 5th edn., Oxford: Blackwell Scientific Publications.

Cannon, W. B. & Rosenblueth, A. (1937) *Autonomic Neuro-Effector Systems*. New York: The Macmillan Company.

Huddart, H. & Hunt, S. (1975) *Visceral Muscle its Structure and Function*. London: Blackie.

Koelle, G. B. (1975) Neurohumoral transmission and the autonomic nervous system. In *The Pharmacological Basis of Therapeutics*, 5th edn., pp 404–444, eds. Goodman, L. S. & Gilman, A. New York: Macmillan Publishing Co.

4

Acetylcholine and parasympathomimetic agents

Acetylcholine is present in a great variety of animal species and also in many plants. In man it is the most widespread neurotransmitter substance so far identified and phylogenetically it is thought to be the most ancient transmitter substance. It is the neurotransmitter released by all postganglionic parasympathetic nerves and by a few postganglionic sympathetic nerves. The actions of acetylcholine released from postganglionic autonomic nerves are mimicked by the alkaloid muscarine and are initiated by combination of acetylcholine with specific structures called muscarinic receptors present on the postsynaptic cells. Other substances, both naturally-occurring and synthetic, also stimulate muscarinic receptors and therefore mimick the effects of parasympathetic nerve stimulation; these substances are called *parasympathomimetics*. A later but less specific term to describe drugs with actions resembling those of acetylcholine is *cholinomimetic*.

SYNTHESIS, STORAGE AND RELEASE OF ACETYLCHOLINE

Acetylcholine is synthesised within cholinergic neurones by the transfer of an acetyl group from acetylcoenzyme A to the organic base choline. A specific enzyme called *choline acetyltransferase (choline acetylase)* is necessary for this reaction to occur (Fig. 4.1). Coenzyme A is widely distributed in the body and choline is an essential dietary constituent being one of the B complex group of vitamins. Choline acetyltransferase is itself synthesised in the cell bodies of cholinergic neurones from where it passes in the axoplasm down the axons towards the nerve endings. A small amount of acetylcholine is produced throughout the neurone but most is formed in specialised vesicles which are mainly accumulated at the nerve endings and in which the greater part of the neuronal acetylcholine is stored. The vesicles, which are 300–600° A in diameter, combine with the membrane of the nerve ending and discharge their content of acetylcholine into the synaptic cleft. This process, which has been called *exocytosis*, occurs continuously in a random fashion and leads to small but measurable electrical changes in the postsynaptic membrane. Under resting conditions insufficient packets or 'quanta' of acetylcholine are released to combine with sufficient postsynaptic receptors to produce an action potential in the postsynaptic membrane and thereby cause a response in the effector tissue. However, when nerve impulses arrive at a nerve

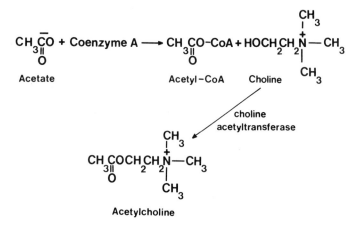

Fig. 4.1 Biosynthesis of acetylcholine.

ending a large number of vesicles simultaneously discharge their content of acetylcholine into the synaptic cleft and sufficient receptors are occupied to cause typical parasympathetic effects in the tissue. Synthesis of acetylcholine within the neurone is in some way controlled by impulses passing down the nerve since it is markedly increased when the frequency of nerve stimulation is increased. Although the precise mechanisms for the synthesis and release of acetylcholine are not fully understood, it seems likely that calcium ions play a major role in the release process since the amount of acetylcholine released from a stimulated cholinergic nerve is proportional to the concentration of calcium ions in the extracellular fluid over a wide range of calcium concentrations. It has been suggested that calcium ions are necessary for the combination of the acetylcholine-containing vesicles with the membrane of the nerve ending.

Hemicholinium (HC-3) and triethylcholine (TEC) are two

substances which induce failure of transmission in cholinergic nerves by interfering with acetylcholine synthesis. It is thought that these substances act by inhibiting the transport of choline across the cell membrane and their effects can be reversed by increasing the extracellular choline concentration. Neither drug is of clinical use but both have been widely used as experimental tools in studies concerned with the mechanisms of acetylcholine synthesis in cholinergic nerves. The release of transmitter from cholinergic nerves is also prevented by the toxin produced by the micro-organism *clostridium botulinum* which is often implicated in cases of food poisoning. Botulinum toxin prevents acetylcholine release by an unknown mechanism which apparently does not involve changes in either the synthesis or storage of acetylcholine.

Combination of acetylcholine with the muscarinic receptor is thought to produce conformational changes in the receptor and/or in the surrounding postsynaptic membrane such that channels open in the membrane through which ions, particularly sodium, can pass and thus produce the electrical changes which take place in the postsynaptic membrane. This activity occurs only in the region of the synapse and is of brief duration being terminated within a few milliseconds by the rapid hydrolysis of acetylcholine molecules, to choline and acetate, by the enzyme *acetylcholinesterase* which in most cholinergic junctions is concentrated in the postsynaptic membrane. The choline released as a result of enzymatic action is partly reabsorbed by the presynaptic terminals for later re-use in acetylcholine production. It is likely that part of the acetylcholine released from nerve endings has its effects terminated by simple diffusion away from the region of the synapse.

The muscarinic receptor

As is the case with other receptors, little is known about the physico-chemical nature of the muscarinic receptor. It is thought likely that it is a water-soluble protein present in the outer lipoprotein layer of the postsynaptic membrane and that its combination with acetylcholine involves spatial fit and electrostatic attraction. The acetylcholine molecule can be thought of as being composed of three parts each of which is involved in the combination with the muscarinic receptor. The quaternised nitrogen atom bearing a strong positive charge is the centre of the so called *cationic head* and gives acetylcholine its basic character. The cationic head is thought to fit into a depression in the receptor surface (the anionic site) which bears a negative electrical charge. Alterations in the acetylcholine molecule which either reduce the charge on the quaternary nitrogen (such as substitution of one or more methyl groups with hydrogen) or increase the size of the cationic head (for instance by replacing the methyl groups with ethyl groups) strongly reduce its muscarinic receptor stimulating potency.

ACETYLCHOLINE MOLECULE

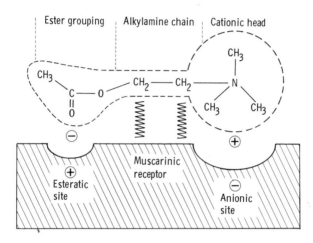

Fig. 4.2 Hypothetical mechanisms involved in the combination of an acetylcholine molecule with a muscarinic receptor.

The *alkylamine chain* is important in providing a bridge of the correct length between the cationic head and the acetyl group of the acetylcholine molecule and thus allowing of simultaneous attachment of both ends of the molecule to the receptor. Increase or decrease in the length of the alkylamine chain markedly reduce the muscarinic stimulant potency of acetylcholine. The alkylamine chain may also aid combination of acetylcholine with the receptor by forming bonds with the receptor via Van de Waals forces.

The acetyl group forms the third important centre of the acetylcholine molecule and bears an overall negative charge. This group is thought to fit into a depression in the receptor surface bearing a positive electrical charge and called the *esteratic site*.

This conceptual picture of the muscarinic receptor (Fig. 4.2) has been of considerable value in the design of new drugs with either stimulant (agonist) or blocking (antagonist) activity on muscarinic receptors. However, it is important to remember that it is only a hypothetical picture and some experimental evidence is not in accord with such a simple explanation of drug/receptor interaction.

PARASYMPATHOMIMETIC DRUGS IN CLINICAL USE

Acetylcholine

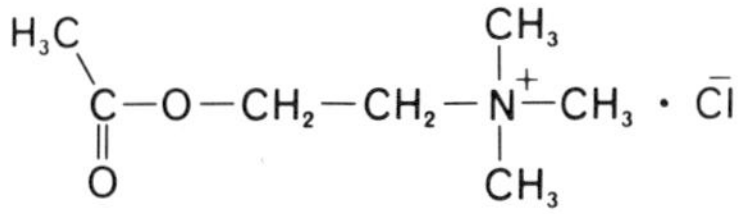

$$H_3C\diagdown \underset{\underset{O}{\|}}{C}-O-CH_2-CH_2-\underset{\underset{CH_3}{|}}{\overset{\overset{CH_3}{|}}{N^+}}-CH_3 \cdot \bar{Cl}$$

acetylcholine chloride

Acetylcholine is the physiological stimulant of both muscarinic and nicotinic receptors and therefore its administration produces widespread, often mutually antagonistic, effects on various organs which are of little clinical use. In addition to this obvious lack of specificity its use as a drug is further limited by its rapid hydrolysis in the body by cholinesterase enzymes and by its total ineffectiveness when given by mouth.

Clinical uses and dosage. Despite its obvious disadvantages acetylcholine does find limited clinical usage when administered by either subcutaneous, intramuscular, intravenous or intra-arterial routes. It has been used intravenously to treat bouts of paroxysmal tachycardia although this route is not without danger due to the cardiac depressant action of acetylcholine and the intramuscular or subcutaneous routes are generally preferred. The dosage by the intramuscular or subcutaneous routes is 20 to 200 mg.

Intra-arterial infusions of up to 100 mg have been recommended to treat vascular occlusion caused by intermittent claudication or the early gangrene of the extremities in diabetic patients.

A 1 per cent solution of acetylcholine chloride with 5 per cent mannitol (MIOCHOL) is used for constricting the pupil during corneal grafting operations.

Methacholine
(acetyl β-methylcholine, methacholine chloride BPC)

$$H_3C \diagdown \underset{\underset{O}{\parallel}}{C} - O - \underset{\underset{CH_3}{|}}{CH} - CH_2 - \underset{\underset{CH_3}{|}}{\overset{\overset{CH_3}{|}}{N^+}} - CH_3 \cdot \overline{Cl}$$

Methacholine only differs from acetylcholine in having a methyl group substituted on the β carbon atom. This slight chemical modification has little effect on the muscarinic receptor stimulant potency of the molecule but virtually abolishes its nicotinic effects. In addition, methacholine is much more slowly hydrolysed by acetylcholinesterase than is acetylcholine and is virtually immune to destruction by the less specific cholinesterases (pseudocholinesterase) of plasma and other tissues. Thus methacholine has more prolonged effects than acetylcholine and is practically specific for muscarinic receptors.

Clinical uses and dosage. Methacholine is used mainly for its effects on the cardiovascular system, particularly for dilating constricted blood vessels in vasospastic conditions of the extremities such as Raynaud's syndrome. It is usually administered for this purpose by the subcutaneous route and in doses of 10 to 25 mg.

It is occasionally administered as a 0·1 to 0·5 per cent aqueous solution by iontophoresis to produce vasodilatation in a restricted area. A subcutaneous dose of 20 mg has been used to treat paroxysmal tachycardia.

All muscarinic receptor stimulant drugs constrict the pupil of the eye and cause spasm of accommodation by constriction of the ciliary muscle. This results in an increased drainage of aqueous humour from the anterior chamber of the eye through the canal of Schlemm. This relieves the increased intra-ocular pressure which occurs in chronic simple glaucoma. Methacholine is sometimes used to treat glaucoma in aqueous solutions containing 2·5 to 20 per cent methacholine but other miotics, especially pilocarpine, are usually preferred for this purpose. Methacholine bromide is less hygroscopic than the chloride and has been used in the USA. to prepare tablets for oral administration. However, the drug is not very active by this route and doses of 200 to 600 mg per day are required.

Carbachol
(carbamoylcholine chloride, carbachol BP.)

$$H_2N-\underset{\underset{O}{\|}}{C}-O-CH_2-CH_2-\underset{\underset{CH_3}{|}}{\overset{\overset{CH_3}{|}}{N^+}}-CH_3 \cdot \bar{C}l$$

Carbachol is derived from acetylcholine by the substitution of an amide group on the acyl carbon atom. This modification renders carbachol immune to hydrolysis by cholinesterase and reduces its nicotinic, but not muscarinic, stimulant potency. Carbachol, therefore, is a potent muscarinic stimulant with a prolonged duration of action and is active orally. Its nicotinic effects, although less than those of acetylcholine, are more pronounced than with any other commonly-used parasympathomimetic.

Clinical uses and dosage. Carbachol is mainly used for its effects in stimulating the intestine and bladder. Orally it is given in daily doses of 1 to 4 mg, although it is mainly used by the subcutaneous route in doses of 250 to 500 micrograms. Carbachol injection BP, BNF contains 250 micrograms per ml.

It is used to treat postoperative intestinal atony and retention of urine. It is also useful for expelling gas from the intestines before X-ray examinations and to speed up the passage of renal stones in the ureters. Like other choline esters it is occasionally used to treat paroxysmal auricular tachycardia. It is used in eye-drops to constrict the pupil and reduce intra-ocular pressure in simple glaucoma. The usual (BPC) concentration of carbachol in eye-drops is 0·8 per cent but concentrations up to 3 per cent may be used.

Bethanechol

$$H_2N-\underset{\underset{O}{\|}}{C}-O-\underset{\underset{CH_3}{|}}{CH}-CH_2-\underset{\underset{CH_3}{|}}{\overset{\overset{CH_3}{|}}{N^+}}-CH_3 \cdot \bar{C}l$$

bethanechol chloride

Bethanechol contains both the amide group of carbachol and the β-methyl group of methacholine. Both substituents help to reduce its nicotinic potency and to render it immune to hydrolysis by cholinesterase making it a long-acting muscarinic stimulant almost devoid of nicotinic activity.

Clinical uses and dosage. Bethanechol is active both by mouth (daily dose 30 to 120 mg) and by the subcutaneous route (dose 2·5 to 30 mg per day). It is used to treat gastric retention following vagotomy, for abdominal distension and for postoperative urinary retention. It is commercially available in the UK as tablets containing 5, 10 or 25 mg (MYOTONINE).

Pilocarpine
(pilocarpine hydrochloride BPC)

$$H_3C-N \overset{CH_2}{\diagdown} CH_2-CH_3 \cdot H\bar{C}l$$

Pilocarpine is a naturally-occurring alkaloid present in the leaflets of the shrub *Maranham jaborandi* which grows in South America. Extracts of the leaves are sometimes added to hair lotions because it has a supposed action in stimulating hair growth.

It is difficult to account for the muscarinic potency of pilocarpine in terms of structure-activity relationships since it bears little resemblance to acetylcholine and does not even contain a quaternary nitrogen which is thought to be a major active centre of the acetylcholine molecule and is present in all the other clinically used choline esters. Pilocarpine has potent muscarinic receptor stimulant potency and much weaker nicotinic activity. It is a particularly potent stimulant of glandular tissues such as sweat and salivary glands.

Clinical uses and dosage. Pilocarpine is not often used by mouth but doses of 2·5 to 5 mg have been recommended for the treatment of constipation, particularly that resulting as a side-effect of treatment with some antihypertensive drugs.

Its main use is for local application to the eye in aqueous solutions containing 1–5 per cent of pilocarpine hydrochloride (BPC, BNF) for the treatment of raised intra-ocular pressure in cases of simple glaucoma and detachment of the retina.

Recently a sustained release formulation of pilocarpine has been introduced for the treatment of glaucoma. In this preparation the active constituent is suspended in an inert plastic matrix which when positioned under the eyelid releases pilocarpine onto the surface of the eye at a rate of either 20 or 40 micrograms per hour (OCUSERT PILO 20 and 40). The plastic insert is normally replaced at weekly intervals.

Contra-indications for the use of parasympathomimetics
Since all the drugs in this class have a basically similar mode of action then the same contra-indications apply to the systemic use of each. All of the major contra-indications of these drugs arise

from their actions in stimulating muscarinic receptors and therefore of mimicking the effects of parasympathetic stimulation. They cause bronchoconstriction and are not therefore used in asthmatic patients since they may provoke an acute attack. They are not used in patients suffering from hyperthyroidism in whom they are particularly likely to cause atrial fibrillation. In patients suffering from myocardial ischaemia their use may further reduce coronary blood flow probably as a result of the lowering of arterial blood pressure which they cause. Finally they are contra-indicated in patients suffering from peptic ulceration because they increase gastric acid secretion.

SUMMARY

Acetylcholine is the neurotransmitter substance released from postganglionic parasympathetic nerve endings; it produces its effects by combining with muscarinic receptors situated on the postsynaptic cells. The combination of acetylcholine molecules with muscarinic receptors is believed to involve spatial 'fit' and electrostatic attraction. Acetylcholine is synthesised in cholinergic nerves by the transfer of an acetyl group from acetyl-coenzyme A to choline in the presence of the enzyme choline acetyltransferase. Acetylcholine is stored intraneuronally in vesicles which, on passage of nerve impulses down the axons, combine with the neuronal membrane and discharge their contents from the nerve endings into the synaptic clefts. After combination with muscarinic receptors acetylcholine is rapidly inactivated by hydrolysis to choline and acetate by the enzyme acetylcholinesterase.

Acetylcholine is little used clinically because of its widespread and transient effects. Methacholine, carbachol and bethanechol are clinically useful choline esters which are more stable to hydrolysis by cholinesterases and which have similar muscarinic, but less nicotinic, actions than acetylcholine. Pilocarpine is a naturally-occurring parasympathomimetic with little structural resemblance to acetylcholine which acts predominantly on muscarinic receptors. The main clinical uses of the parasympathomimetic drugs are to increase the tone and motility of the intestine and bladder in atonic states, to dilate blood vessels in vasospastic conditions and to constrict the pupil and reduce intra-ocular pressure in simple glaucoma. These drugs are contra-indicated in patients suffering from asthma, hyperthyroidism, myocardial ischaemia and peptic ulceration.

GENERAL READING

Barlow, R. B. (1964) *Introduction to Chemical Pharmacology*. London: Menthuen & Co. Ltd.

Bebbington, A. & Brimblecombe, R. W. (1965) Muscarinic receptors in the peripheral and central nervous systems, *Adv. Drug. Res.*, **2**, 143–172.

Bowman, W. C., Rand, M. J. & West, G. B. (1968) *Textbook of Pharmacology*, Oxford: Blackwell Scientific Publications.

Carrier, O. (1972) *Pharmacology of the Peripheral Autonomic Nervous System*, Chicago: Year Book Medical Publishers Inc.

Huddart, H. & Hunt, S. (1975) *Visceral Muscle its Structure and Function*, London: Blackie.

Koelle, G. B. (1975) Parasympathomimetic agents. In *The Pharmacological Basis of Therapeutics*, 5th edn., pp 467–476, Goodman, L. S. & Gilman, A., eds. New York: Macmillan Publishing Co.

Martindale (1977) *The Extra Pharmacopoeia* 27th edn., London: The Pharmaceutical Press.

Triggle, D. J. (1965) *Chemical Aspects of the Autonomic Nervous System*. London: Academic Press.

5

Anticholinesterase agents

The cholinesterases are a group of enzymes which share the common property of hydrolysing ester bonds but differ in their substrate specificity. The cholinesterase found largely in the postsynaptic membranes at cholinergic synapses is called *acetylcholinesterase* (sometimes also referred to as true or specific cholinesterase); its function is to rapidly terminate the activity of acetylcholine released from cholinergic nerve endings. Red blood cells are another rich source of acetylcholinesterase but its function at this site is unknown. Another group of cholinesterases, collectively called non-specific or *pseudocholinesterase*, is found in plasma, intestine and to a lesser extent in other tissues. The functions of pseudocholinesterase are not clear but it has been suggested that in the intestine it is involved in regulating the proposed action of acetylcholine in controlling rhythmic movements and tone of the intestine. The substrate specificity of acetylcholinesterase differs from that of pseudo-cholinesterase. Thus methacholine is hydrolysed by acetyl-cholinesterase but not by pseudocholinesterase and the reverse is true of succinylcholine, a choline ester which finds clinical use as a skeletal muscle relaxant. However, both types of enzyme readily hydrolyse acetylcholine. Most studies have been concerned with actions of acetylcholinesterase since it appears that most clinical use can be made of its inhibition.

INTERACTION OF ACETYLCHOLINE WITH ACETYLCHOLINESTERASE

The combination of an acetylcholine molecule with a cholinesterase molecule is believed to closely resemble the combination of acetylcholine with the muscarinic receptor described in the previous chapter.. Like the muscarinic receptor, the cholinesterase molecule is believed to have two active sites (esteratic and anionic) for combination with the acetylcholine molecules.

Combination of the positively charged cationic head of acetyl-choline with the negatively charged anionic site of cholinesterase is believed to anchor and orientate the acetylcholine molecule such that the ester linkage may be broken. The acetyl group of acetylcholine is then thought to combine with cholinesterase via formation of a covalent bond with the esterastic site of cholin-esterase. The hydrolysis of acetylcholine molecules takes place in three stages (Fig. 5.1). First, acetylcholine and cholinesterase form an equilibrium complex. This is followed by rupture of the ester linkage of acetylcholine and release of choline to leave an acetylated form of cholinesterase. In the final stage the acetyl-enzyme reacts with water to form acetic acid and to leave a regenerated cholinesterase molecule ready to enter into combin-ation with a further molecule of acetylcholine.

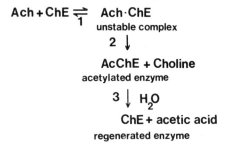

Fig. 5.1 The hydrolysis of acetylcholine (Ach) by acetylcholinesterase (ChE); (1) formation of equilibrium complex; (2) release of choline from the complex to leave acetylated enzyme and (3) removal of water to leave regenerated enzyme.

Anticholinesterase agents have been developed which prevent the hydrolysis of acetylcholine by cholinesterase by forming a stable complex with cholinesterase and thus competing with acetylcholine for occupation of the active sites of cholinesterase. This type of enzyme inhibition is known as competitive in-hibition. Anticholinesterases by delaying the destruction of nervously-released acetylcholine produce widespread effects in the body due to enhancement of the effects of cholinergic nerve stimulation. Thus they will modify transmission in autonomic ganglia, at postganglionic parasympathetic nerve endings, at the junctions of somatic nerves with voluntary muscles and, with some agents, at synapses within the central nervous system. One group of clinical uses for anticholinesterases is based on their actions in increasing the effects produced by parasympathetic stimulation and thus in this respect these drugs have the same indications and uses as the parasympathomimetic substances which directly stimulate muscarinic receptors (see Fig. 5.2). The other main uses of anticholinesterases is based on their effects in inhibiting acetylcholinesterase at the junction of somatic nerves with skeletal (voluntary) muscle. At this site anticholinesterases are used to antagonise the actions of muscle relaxant drugs such as d-tubocurarine which compete with acetylcholine for the

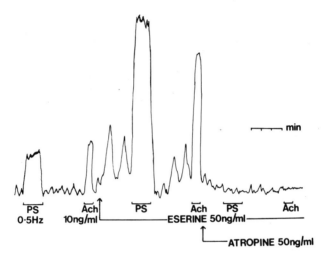

Fig. 5.2 Pharmacological effects of eserine and atropine.

An isolated strip of smooth muscle from a rat stomach suspended in Kreb's solution contracted when the parasympathetic nerve endings in the tissue were electrically stimulated (PS) and when acetylcholine (Ach) was added to the bath. Both responses were greatly increased in the presence of eserine but were abolished after the further addition of atropine.

occupation of nicotinic receptors in skeletal muscle and which are widely used during surgical procedures. The anticholinesterases are also useful in the diagnosis and treatment of myasthenia gravis, a condition in which there is weakness of voluntary muscles due to deficient production of acetylcholine by the cholinergic nerves.

The anticholinesterase drugs are classified into two groups, reversible and irreversible, depending on the rate at which cholinesterase is regenerated after inhibition. In general, the reversible anticholinesterases are of most clinical value but the irreversible inhibitors have been made on a large scale for use as insecticides and for potential use in warfare as 'nerve gases' and to a much lesser extent for use as therapeutic agents.

Reversible anticholinesterases

Physostigmine
(eserine)

Historically physostigmine was the first anticholinesterase to be discovered and used clinically. It also has an important place in the history of the development of the theory of neurohumoral transmission since it has been widely used to protect acetyl-choline released from cholinergic nerve endings in many experimental situations. Physostigmine occurs naturally in Calabar beans obtained from the plant *Physostigma venenosum* which is indigenous to tropical West Africa. The beans which somewhat resemble broad beans in appearance contain 0·04 to 0·3 per cent physostigmine in the cotyledons, and have been used probably for centuries in tribal trials by ordeal. The basis of this primitive system of justice was (and probably is) that a person or persons suspected of having committed a crime were required to eat some Calabar beans (locally called 'ordeal' beans). If the suspects died from the widespread pharmacological effects of the beans (as most did) they were deemed to have been guilty of the crime. Survival of the 'ordeal' was sometimes achieved by 'innocent' persons who were fortunate enough to vomit before they absorbed a lethal dose of physostigmine. Calabar beans were brought to England in 1840 and the pure alkaloid was isolated in 1864 by Jobst & Hesse who named it physostigmine. The following year Vee & Leven (1865) isolated the same alkaloid which they called eserine. Curiously, both names have survived to the present day.

Physostigmine contains tertiary nitrogen atoms which at bodily pH exist in the positively charged cationic form and thus combine with the negatively charged anionic site of cholinesterase. When given by mouth the drug is rapidly absorbed from the gastrointestinal tract and its actions in the body are terminated by dissociation of the drug-enzyme complex as the extracellular level of drug falls and also by the slow hydrolysis of the ester linkage of physostigmine by cholinesterase. In practice, physostigmine is rarely used systematically, its use now being almost entirely restricted to local application to the eye.

Clinical uses and dosage. Physostigmine salicylate BP may be administered orally in doses of 0·5 to 1 mg with a maximum recommended dosage of 3 mg in 24 hours, or by intra-muscular injection in a dose of 500 micrograms. Its main systemic use is in the treatment of atropine poisoning in which it has the advantage over many other anticholinesterases in that it readily crosses the blood/brain barrier and will therefore antagonise central as well as peripheral effects of atropine.

It finds occasional use to stimulate the intestine and bladder in atonic states but neostigmine is usually preferred in these conditions.

The main clinical use of physostigmine at the present time is in the form of eye-drops for use as a miotic to treat glaucoma. In general, the anticholinesterases produce a more persistent lowering of intra-ocular pressure in simple glaucoma than do parasympathomimetics such as pilocarpine. Preparations in common use are Physostigmine Eye-Drops (BPC, BNF) which contains 0·25 or 0·5 per cent physostigmine sulphate and Physostigmine and Pilocarpine Eye-Drops (BPC, BNF) which usually contains 0·25 or 0·5 per cent physostigmine sulphate with 2 or 4 per cent pilocarpine hydrochloride. Physostigmine sulphate is preferred to the salicylate in eye-drop preparations because it is more soluble in water and is compatible with a wider range of preservatives. However, all aqueous solutions of physostigmine are more or less unstable and with time coloured oxidation products form especially in the presence of light.

Physostigmine eye-drops form a useful means of antagonising the mydriatic effect of atropine or related substances used in ophthalmic investigations.

Neostigmine

Neostigmine is a synthetic quaternary ammonium compound with a rapid onset of action and similar anticholinesterase activity to physostigmine. It differs from physostigmine in that it is poorly absorbed by mouth and has somewhat stronger effects at nicotinic sites.

Clinical uses and dosage. Neostigmine is most widely used for its effects at nicotinic sites to terminate the skeletal muscle relaxant effect of d-tubocurarine and related drugs and in the treatment of myasthenia gravis. As an anti-curare neostigmine is administered as the methylsulphate by either intramuscular or subcutaneous injection. The official (BP, BNF) injection contains 500 micrograms in 1 ml and the usual dose is 0·5 to 2 mg. In the treatment of myasthenia gravis, unwanted autonomic side effects of neostigmine may be abolished by atropine. In myasthenia neostigmine may be given by injection or, more conveniently, orally (dose 15 to 30 mg repeated 3 or 4 times daily). The official (BP, BNF) tablets of neostigmine each contain 15 mg of neostigmine bromide.

The conditions of the autonomic system in which neostigmine is used include atonic conditions of the intestine and bladder, chronic constipation in children, expulsion of ureteric calculi and expulsion of intestinal gas prior to X-ray examination to facilitate visualisation of organs such as the gall-bladder, kidneys, ureters and intestine. Neostigmine (as a 3–5 per cent aqueous solution) finds occasional use for instillation into the eye in the treatment of glaucoma.

Neostigmine may also be used to differentiate between delayed menstruation and pregnancy. For this use it is injected intramuscularly in a dose of 1 mg on each of three successive days. In cases of delayed menstruation it will initiate bleeding within 3 days but will have no such effect in pregnancy.

In addition to the official (BP, BNF) preparations neostigmine is also available as tablets, injection and ophthalmic solution under the trade-name of PROSTIGMIN.

Pyridostigmine (Pyridostigmine Bromide B.P.)

Chemically and pharmacologically this substance is closely related to neostigmine. It has a slower onset and a slightly longer duration of action than neostigmine but offers little practical advantage over it in clinical use.

Clinical uses and dosage. Its clinical indications are as for neostigmine. It is available as official (BP, BNF) tablets containing 60 mg pyridostigmine bromide and an injection (BP) containing 1 mg in 1 ml, and as proprietary preparations (MESTINON) of the same strength. The usual dosage is 60 to

240 mg orally or 1 to 5 mg by intramuscular or subcutaneous injection.

Benzpyrinium

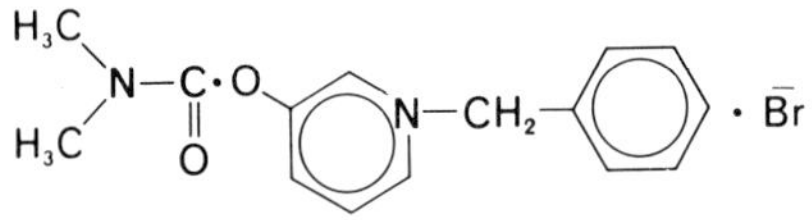

This is another neostigmine analogue which finds occasional use to treat atonic states of the bowel and bladder and in the treatment of simple delayed menstruation. Doses up to 2 mg are used by intramuscular injection.

Distigmine

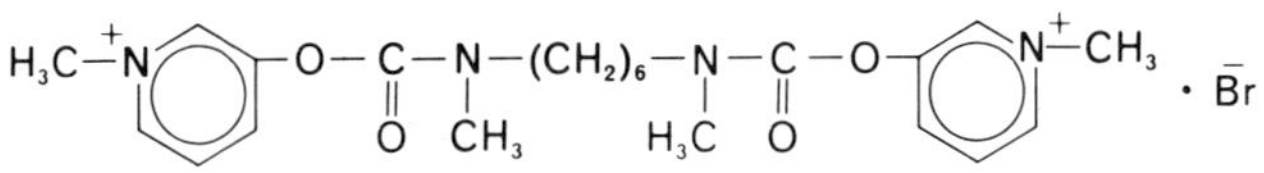

Distigmine differs from neostigmine in having a longer duration of action, its effects lasting at least 24 hours. It is used to treat atonic conditions of the bladder and bowel and treatment may need to be repeated as infrequently as every third day. The usual dose is 5 mg orally or 500 micrograms by intramuscular injection. It is commercially available (UBRETID) as tablets containing 5 mg and an injection containing 500 micrograms in 1 ml.

Demecarium (Bis-neostigmine bromide)

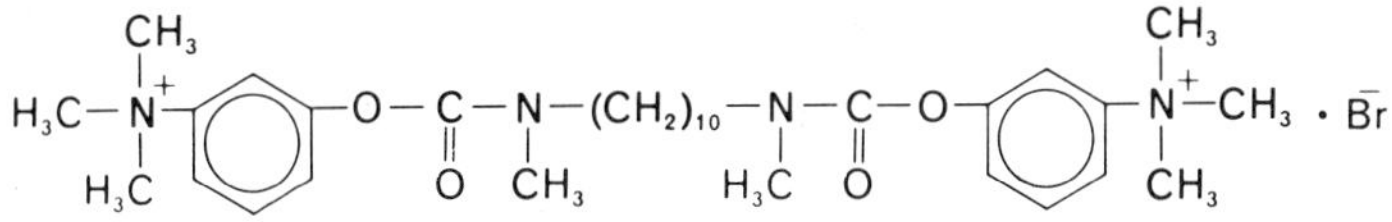

This compound consists of two neostigmine molecules joined by a chain of 10 methylene (CH_2) groups. It is somewhat more potent than neostigmine and has a very prolonged effect. Its main use is in the management of glaucoma where its miotic effect is evident within 20 minutes of instillation into the eye and may persist for a week or more. The usual dosage in glaucoma is from 2 drops of a 0·25 per cent solution instilled twice weekly to 1 to 2 drops twice daily. Demecarium is also used in the management of accommodative convergent strabismus (esotropia), a type of squint which particularly affects children.

Demecarium is commercially available as eye-drops containing 0·25 or 0·5 per cent in aqueous solution (TOSMILEN).

Two other reversible anticholinesterases which are used clinically are ambenonium chloride (MYTELASE) and edrophonium chloride (TENSILON). However, these compounds are not used for their autonomic effects. Ambenonium is given orally in the treatment of myasthenia gravis and edrophonium, which has a very brief duration of action, is used in the diagnosis of the same condition.

Irreversible anticholinesterases

These substances, which are mainly organic compounds containing pentavalent phosphorus, are extremely long-acting and potent anticholinesterases. A great amount of research effort has been devoted to the synthesis of this series of compounds and it has been estimated that at least 50 000 different compounds have been prepared. Much of this work has been performed by Schrader and his group in Germany. Schrader (1952) suggested the following general formula for the series:

$$\begin{array}{c} R_1 \\ \diagdown \\ P = O \, (\text{or S}) \\ \diagup \diagdown \\ R_2 X \end{array}$$

Many organophosphorus compounds do not have a quaternised nitrogen to react with the negatively charged anionic site of cholinesterase and these substances are thought to react only with the esteratic site of cholinesterase. The stages in the interaction of these compounds with cholinesterase are generally similar to that of the reversible inhibitors. The inhibitor and enzyme at first enter into a complex which is still capable of dissociation; this is followed by removal by hydrolysis of the group X from the inhibitor leaving the esteratic site of cholinesterase phosphorylated. Unlike the complex formed between the reversible inhibitors and cholinesterase the phosphorylated form of cholinesterase is extremely stable and removal of the phosphoryl group from the enzyme may take weeks or months and thus for most practical purposes is irreversible. The very long duration of action of these substances coupled with their extreme potency make them potentially extremely toxic. The toxicity is further accentuated by the ease with which they are absorbed by mouth, inhalation and even by skin contact and by their lipid solubility which enables them to pass readily into the central nervous system.

Inhibition of cholinesterase enzymes has proved to be a very effective way of killing insects and the organophosphorus compounds have been widely used for this purpose. However, considerable precautions are necessary for the safe handling of these compounds and there have been a number of fatal accidents to agricultural workers arising from their use. The compounds have also been made in large quantities by some governments for potential use in chemical warfare. These substances include the 'nerve gases' tabun, sarin and soman which are among the most toxic synthetic substances that man's ingenuity has thus far led him to produce. Many members of this class of compound are chemically very stable so the disposal of unwanted stocks create great problems and provide a toxic hazard for this and future generations.

In general, the organophosphorus compounds are too toxic for routine clinical use but some members of the group find a limited clinical usage in conditions such as glaucoma where their prolonged effects may be an advantage.

Dyflos (Di-isopropylfluorophosphonate, DFP)

DFP is a clear liquid which forms unstable solutions in water and is only used clinically dissolved in arachis oil. It inhibits pseudocholinesterase before acetylcholinesterase and its duration of action is of the order of 10 days.

Clinical uses and dosage. DFP is used by topical application to the conjunctiva in the treatment of glaucoma. It is administered usually as a 0·1 per cent solution in arachis oil and is generally only resorted to when other miotics have failed. The usual dose is one drop instilled once or twice daily. It may prevent focussing of the eye by causing ciliary spasm and the inconvenience of this can be lessened by using the eye-drops at night.

A 0·025 per cent solution is occasionally used in the treatment of esotropia.

Escothiopate (Escothiopate Iodide)

$$C_2H_5O \diagdown \hspace{-0.3em} \underset{C_2H_5O \diagup}{\overset{\displaystyle O}{P}} \diagdown SCH_2 \cdot CH_2 \cdot \overset{\displaystyle CH_3}{\underset{\displaystyle CH_3}{N}} \hspace{-0.3em}{}^{+}\hspace{-0.3em}-CH_3 \cdot \bar{I}'$$

Escothiopate has the advantage over Dyflos in that it forms stable solutions in water and thus obviates the need for oily eye-drops which some patients find uncomfortable to use. It has a very prolonged effect and when instilled into the eye produces a miotic effect within 10 to 45 minutes which may persist for one to four weeks.

Clinical uses and dosage. The official preparation (Escothiopate Eye-Drops, BNF) contain 0.06, 0.125 or 0.25 per cent escothiopate iodide in aqueous solution. The usual dose in the treatment of glaucoma is one drop once or twice daily. Eye-drops containing 0.25 per cent escothiopate may be used for short periods in the treatment of esotropia. Proprietary preparations of escothiopate are marketed under the trade-name of PHOSPHOLINE IODIDE.

Toxic effects of anticholinesterase therapy

In general, the same contra-indications apply to anticholinesterases as to parasympathomimetics. Thus they may induce bronchoconstriction and may therefore provoke acute attacks in asthmatic patients. They should also be used with caution in patients suffering from either cardiac ischaemia or gastric ulceration.

In cases of overdosage with anticholinesterases the autonomic effects can usually be controlled by atropine. In the case of overdosage with organophosphorus compounds certain compounds have been developed which are able to regenerate the inhibited cholinesterase by removal of the phosphoryl group. These compounds are all strongly basic and have a positively charged quaternary nitrogen atom. The best known of these cholinesterase regenerators is *pralidoxime* (pyridine-2-aldoxime methiodide, P_2-AM). These agents are most effective if administered without delay after the organophosphorus compound since the phosphoryl group becomes more difficult to remove with time. Atropine is also useful in the treatment of poisoning by organophosphorus compounds and may be used in combination with substances such as pralidoxime.

Recent evidence strongly suggests that treatment of glaucoma with potent anticholinesterase agents such as demecarium, escothiopate and DFP for periods longer than 6 months carries a high risk of cataract formation especially in elderly patients. It also seems that pilocarpine does not carry this risk and pharmaceutical research, which has culminated in the introduction of sustained release preparations of pilocarpine, holds out hope of a safer treatment for this condition in the future.

SUMMARY

The physiological effects of acetylcholine in the body are terminated by hydrolysis of the ester linkage of the molecule by the enzyme *acetylcholinesterase*. Another group of similar enzymes, collectively called *pseudocholinesterase*, is present in the plasma, gut and in some other tissues. The physiological function of pseudocholinesterase has yet to be established with certainty. Combination of acetylcholine with acetylcholinesterase is believed to involve similar spatial and electrostatic factors as does combination of acetylcholine molecules with muscarinic receptors. Compounds have been developed *(anticholinesterases)* which compete with acetylcholine for the active sites of acetylcholinesterase but which inhibit the enzyme by forming more stable complexes with it. Anticholinesterases may produce widespread effects in the body by increasing the effectiveness of acetylcholine released by cholinergic nerves in the autonomic nervous system, in voluntary muscle and, with some compounds, in the central nervous system. These drugs are divided into two groups, reversible and irreversible, according to the stability of the complex formed with acetylcholinesterase. The reversible inhibitors which include physostigmine, neostigmine and demecarium are used clinically to treat atonic states of the gastrointestinal tract and bladder and to reduce intra-ocular pressure in glaucoma. Some members of this group are also used to antagonise the effects of muscle relaxants of the d-tubocurarine type and to increase voluntary muscle strength in myasthenia gravis.

The irreversible anticholinesterases are mostly organophosphorus compounds which produce a very stable phosphorylated form of acetylcholinesterase. These substances are highly toxic and are widely used as insecticides and have been developed for use in warfare. Two members of this group, dyflos and escothiopate, are used clinically in the treatment of glaucoma.

Poisoning by organophosphorus compounds may be treated with basic substances such as pralidoxime which displace the phosphoryl group from the phosphorylated enzyme and also by repeated administration of atropine.

REFERENCES

Jobst, J. & Hesse, O. (1864) Uber die bohne von calabar. *Ann. der Chem. und Pharm.*, **129**, 115–121.

Schrader, G. (1952) *Die Entwicklung neuer Insektizide auf Grundlage von Organischen Fluor-und Phosphorverbindungen.* Monographie No. 62, Weinheim: Verlag Chemie.

Vee, M. & Leven, M. (1865) De l'alcaloide de la fève de Calabar et expériences physiologiques avec ce même alcaloide. *J. Pharm. et Chimie*, **1**, 70–72.

GENERAL READING

Bowman, W. C., Rand, M. J. & West, G. B. (1968) *Textbook of Pharmacology.* Oxford:Blackwell Scientific Publications.

Brimblecombe, R. W. (1974) *Drug Actions on Cholinergic Systems.* London: The Macmillan Press Ltd.

Karczmar, A. G. (Ed.) (1970) Anticholinesterase agents. In *International Encyclopedia of Pharmacology and Therapeutics*, Section 13, vol. 1. Oxford: Pergamon Press.

Koelle, G. B. (1975) Anticholinesterase agents, In *The Pharmacological Basis of Therapeutics*, 5th edn., pp 445–466, (eds.) Goodman, L. S. & Gilman, A. New York: Macmillan Publishing Co.

6

Muscarinic receptor blocking agents (antimuscarinics)

Atropine is the classical antagonist for the effects produced by drugs which stimulate acetylcholine receptors of the muscarinic type. Dale (1914) classified as muscarinic those actions of acetylcholine which were mimicked by muscarine and abolished by atropine. Acetylcholine released from all postganglionic parasympathetic, and from some postganglionic sympathetic, nerves produces its characteristic effects by reversibly combining with muscarinic receptors present in the postsynaptic cells. It is evident that some muscarinic receptors are not associated directly with nerve endings since acetylcholine and other muscarinic receptor stimulants produce effects in tissues, for instance some blood vessels, which do not receive a parasympathetic innervation. Atropine is a highly specific and persistent antagonist of the effects produced by muscarinic receptor stimulation whether induced by acetylcholine released from parasympathetic nerves or by administration of parasympathomimetic drugs. However, like many other receptor antagonists, atropine is often somewhat less effective in blocking the effects of acetylcholine released from parasympathetic nerve endings than it is in blocking the effects of exogenously administered parasympathomimetic substances. The reason for this is not entirely clear but some possible explanations will be mentioned later in this chapter.

Terminology. Various terms have been used to describe the actions of atropine and related substances; they include parasympatholytic, spasmolytic and anticholinergic. These terms are not sufficiently precise and may be misleading; the terms which will be used in this monograph are muscarinic receptor blocking agent or antimuscarinic.

ATROPINE AND HYOSCINE

Occurrence. Atropine and hyoscine are examples of naturally-occurring plant bases called alkaloids. Both chemically and pharmacologically the substances are closely related and their properties will be discussed together. Both substances occur in members of the Solanaceae family of plants, members of which have been used medicinally for many hundreds of years. The plants which have been most extensively utilized are *Atropa belladonna* (deadly nightshade), *Hyoscyamus niger* (black henbane) and *Datura strammonium* (thorn apple). The main alkaloids present in these plants are hyoscyamine and hyoscine.

Historical notes concerning the medicinal use of solanaceous plants. Solanaceous plants have been used in medicine for at least two thousand years. Deadly nightshade gained popularity

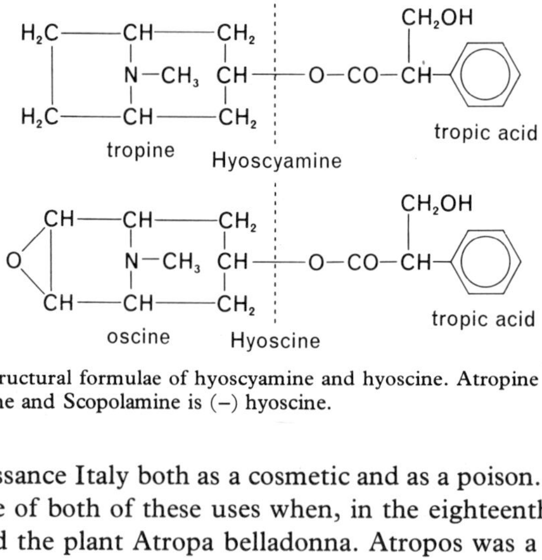

Fig. 6.1 Structural formulae of hyoscyamine and hyoscine. Atropine is ($\pm$) hyoscyamine and Scopolamine is ($-$) hyoscine.

in Renaissance Italy both as a cosmetic and as a poison. Linnaeus took note of both of these uses when, in the eighteenth century, he named the plant Atropa belladonna. Atropos was a female of Greek mythology, eldest of the three Fates, whose task it was to cut the thread of life, whilst belladonna in Italian means 'beautiful woman' an allusion to the use of the plant for making extracts which when instilled into the eyes make the pupils larger and the eyes more attractive. Belladonna extracts became popular in European medicine about the middle of the nineteenth century but the use of atropine as premedication before surgery did not become widespread until the 1920's.

The alkaloids are optically active, the laevo ($-$) isomers being at least twenty times more active than the dextro ($+$) isomers. Hyoscyamine occurs in nature mainly as the ($-$) isomer but racemisation occurs during extraction and atropine is the racemic mixture ($\pm$) hyoscyamine. Hyoscine, which is also called scopolamine, is ($-$) hyoscine. Atropine was first isolated in a pure form by Mein (1833) and its characteristic effect in blocking responses to parasympathetic nerve stimulation was described by Bezold & Bloebaum (1867) and was subsequently confirmed by many workers including Langley and Dale who both used it in early experiments concerning the neurohumoral theory of nerve transmission and the classification of acetylcholine receptors.

Combination of atropine and hyoscine with muscarinic receptors

Atropine and hyoscine exhibit a high degree of stereo-specificity in their antimuscarinic effects and the conclusion which has been generally drawn from this is that there exist at least three points of attachment between the antagonist molecules and the muscarinic receptor. The nitrogen atom is one likely point of attachment since at physiological pH it is ionized, bears a positive charge and may become attached to the negatively charged anionic site of the muscarinic receptor. The other likely active sites of the atropine/hyoscine molecule are the hydroxyl group and the benzene ring of the tropic acid moeity. If the tropine and tropic acid parts of the molecule are separated by hydrolysis then the individual components have virtually no antimuscarinic activity indicating the importance of the ester linkage to the activity of the whole molecule. Reduction of the nitrogen group from tertiary to secondary reduces the positive charge on the nitrogen atom and also the antimuscarinic potency of the molecule. Conversely, increasing the extent of the positive charge on the nitrogen atom by quaternisation increases anti-muscarinic activity but only at the expense of some loss of specificity since these compounds also have significant blocking action on the nicotinic receptors of autonomic ganglia.

The antimuscarinic activity of atropine and hyoscine are a consequence of their prolonged occupation of acetylcholine receptors of the muscarinic type which prevents access of acetylcholine, or similar agonists, to active sites of the muscarinic receptor. The antagonism of the effects of muscarinic receptor stimulation by atropinic drugs is of the competitive (also called surmountable) type since it can be reversed by increasing the concentration of muscarinic receptor agonist in the region of the receptors. This fact is of importance both clinically and experimentally and the most effective way of reversing the effects of atropinic drugs is to increase the concentration of acetylcholine at the receptor site by preventing the action of cholinesterases in destroying the acetylcholine released from cholinergic nerves. Thus anticholinesterase drugs and atropine produce mutually antagonistic effects on the autonomic nervous system (see Fig. 5.2) and this fact is utilised in cases of poisoning by either agent.

Pharmacological effects of atropine and hyoscine

The peripheral effects of hyoscine and atropine are very similar and, in general, are predictable from a knowledge of the functioning of the autonomic nervous system.

Cardiovascular system

The main effect of full muscarinic receptor blocking doses of atropine in man and higher animals is an increase in heart rate (tachycardia) brought about by blockade of the inhibitory influence of the parasympathetic (vagi) nerves to the heart leaving sympathetic effects unopposed. The tachycardia is sometimes preceded by a brief bradycardia which is believed to be due to a transient stimulation of the vagal centre in the medulla. The extent of the tachycardia varies in different individuals according to the resting level of parasympathetic activity ('vagal tone'). In general, atropine produces a marked tachycardia in young adults where vagal tone is high and has relatively little effect in children or in the elderly, both of which groups have low vagal tone. In healthy young adults a full blocking dose of atropine (about 2 mg) may double the resting heart rate to levels around 150 beats per minute. Hyoscine is approximately equipotent with atropine in blocking cardiac muscarinic receptors but in man it usually causes bradycardia rather than tachycardia. The reason for this interesting difference between the actions of atropine and hyoscine is not known. The changes in heart rate produced by atropine and hyoscine are not usually accompanied by any significant changes in the level of arterial blood pressure owing to the influence of cardiovascular reflexes which maintain cardiac output at a virtually unchanged level.

Atropine and hyoscine have little effect on the calibre of blood vessels since most vessels do not receive any significant innervation from the parasympathetic system. However, the blood vessels serving some skeletal muscles are innervated by cholinergic sympathetic fibres which induce vasodilatation during exercise. The vasodilator effects of stimulating these nerves are blocked by atropine in both human and animal studies. However, in man, atropine produces little effect on skeletal muscle blood flow during exercise since it appears that locally produced metabolites of muscular activity are more important in producing vasodilatation than are cholinergic nerves. In large doses atropine causes profound vasodilatation of the superficial skin vessels of the face and neck giving rise to a deeply flushed appearance ('atropine flush'). This effect is apparently unrelated to the antimuscarinic effects of atropine and has occasionally resulted in the effects of atropine-poisoning in children being confused with the symptoms of scarlet fever.

Gastrointestinal system

Atropine, although very effective in preventing the effects of parasympathomimetic and anticholinesterase drugs in stimulating increases in gastrointestinal motility and secretion, is much less effective in antagonising the effects of parasympathetic (vagal) stimulation. In man atropine reduces gastrointestinal motility but does not abolish it even at very high doses. This may be due to the presence of atropine-resistant cholinergic neurones in the wall of the gut and possibly also due to the involvement in gut movements of neurones releasing transmitters (as yet not positively identified) other than acetylcholine. Atropine and hyoscine appear to have an effect on the tone and motility of intestinal smooth muscle, particularly when this is abnormally high, which may be unrelated to muscarinic receptor blockade. This direct effect is sometimes referred to as an 'antispasmodic' action and is a property shared by a number of other compounds some of which, like atropine and hyoscine, possess local anaesthetic activity.

In man, both atropine and hyoscine reduce the secretion of saliva from the parasympathetically-innervated salivary glands but neither affects the accompanying vasodilatation which is now known to be caused mainly by the local release of bradykinin, a polypeptide with vasodilator activity. In man, usual doses of atropine (up to 1 mg) do not produce marked effects on gastric secretion whereas higher doses reduce the volume but not necessarily the acid content of the gastric fluid. Thus, the fasting secretion of gastric acid in man may be almost abolished by a full blocking dose of atropine whereas the quantity released during the psychic and gastric phase of secretion may be virtually unchanged. The duration of action of atropine on gastric secretion is brief when compared with the prolonged inhibition of salivary secretion which it causes. Atropine has little effect on other secretions of the gastrointestinal tract such as pancreatic juice and bile. These facts together underline the relatively greater importance of hormonal rather than neural mechanisms in the control of gastrointestinal secretions.

Secretory glands

The effects of atropine and hyoscine on the secretion of saliva and gastrointestinal juices has already been mentioned. These substances also inhibit the secretion of other glands normally activated by the parasympathetic system. Thus they decrease the secretion of mucus from the glands lining the respiratory tract resulting in drying of the mucous membranes lining the mouth, nose, pharynx and bronchi. The eccrine sweat glands of the skin are innervated by cholinergic sympathetic fibres which are also blocked by antimuscarinic substances leading to a dry skin. Large doses of these drugs completely inhibit sweating which in turn leads to an increase in body temperature; an effect most noticeable in children. In general, hyoscine is rather more potent than atropine in inhibiting secretions from parasympathetically-innervated glands.

Urinary tract

In man, atropine and hyoscine relax the detrusor muscle of the bladder but the contractions of the bladder in response to parasympathetic (pelvic nerve) stimulation are only partly inhibited. Both drugs also decrease the tone and amplitude of the contractions of the ureters.

Respiratory tract

The smooth muscle of the bronchi and bronchioles receive parasympathetic nerves which, when stimulated, contract the muscle and constrict the airway. Atropine and hyoscine, by abolishing parasympathetic tone, cause a relaxation of the bronchi and bronchioles resulting in a widening of the airway.

The eye

Atropine and hyoscine abolish the effects of parasympathetic stimulation to the smooth muscle of the pupil and to the ciliary muscle attached to the lens. This results in dilatation of the pupil (mydriasis) and paralysis of accommodation (cycloplegia). The lens is focussed for distant vision and the pupillary reflex constrictions normally occurring in bright light or on convergence of the eyes are abolished. The widely dilated pupil may lead to unpleasant sensations in bright light (photophobia). The effects of these drugs on the eye in man appear both after systemic or local application. Instillation of a solution of either drug into the eye may lead to very prolonged effects; complete recovery of accommodation and of the pupillary light reflex may be delayed for 10 days or more.

Atropine and hyoscine have little effect on the intra-ocular pressure of young adults with normal eyes. However, in patients over 40 years of age or in those with raised intra-ocular pressure or with a predisposition toward it, then these drugs may cause an acute increase in intra-ocular pressure. This is caused by the contraction of the iris into the angle of the anterior chamber of the eye blocking drainage of aqueous humour. This raised intra-ocular pressure may precipitate an attack of glaucoma especially in the elderly. Although their spectra of activity on the structures of the eye are identical hyoscine is more potent than atropine on this organ and is generally used in lower concentrations.

Uterus

Atropine and hyoscine have virtually no effect on the contractions of the human uterus. They are therefore of little value in the treatment of painful menstruation but may be used safely during parturition where their effects on the central nervous system of the mother may be useful.

Central nervous system

It is in this system that the most marked differences in the pharmacological effects of atropine and hyoscine occur. In the usual human doses (up to 1 mg) atropine produces no marked effects on the brain. However, larger doses produce marked central stimulation which may cause restlessness, irritability, disorientation, hallucinations and delirium. These effects are all prominent in cases of poisoning with solanaceous alkaloids and the stimulant effects are followed by widespread depression leading eventually to fatal respiratory paralysis. Hyoscine, in contrast, produces only central depression and it is mildly sedative even in therapeutic doses.

Resistance of some tissues to atropine and hyoscine

As previously mentioned the effects produced by parasympathomimetic substances, including acetylcholine, added extrinsically, are in many tissues more readily blocked than are similar responses in the same tissues produced by parasympathetic nerve stimulation. Various explanations have been proposed to explain this phenomenon which in the case of the bladder is very marked. One theory is that receptor blocking drugs such as atropine are bulky molecules and it may be physically difficult for an adequate concentration of them to accumulate in the synaptic cleft in some tissues. Another possibility is that the receptors mainly involved in the responses to nerve stimulation are in close proximity to the nerve terminals whilst extrinsically added drugs may act on other receptors widely distributed in the tissue, some of which are not normally activated by neurally-released transmitter. Thus nerve stimulation might lead to a very high local concentration of acetylcholine at the receptors close to the nerve endings such that the antagonist at these sites becomes relatively ineffective. For such a possibility to hold it follows that the disposition of muscarinic receptors in various tissues must be very different in order to account for the marked atropine-resistance of the bladder on the one hand, and the marked sensitivity of the secretory response of the salivary glands on the other. A further possibility is that one or more substances other than acetylcholine are released by parasympathetic stimulation and that these may produce some of the effects usually ascribed to acetylcholine. This explanation has been shown to be true for the atropine-resistant vasodilatation in the salivary glands which accompanies parasympathetic stimulation and which has been shown to be due to the release of the polypeptide substance bradykinin.

Absorption and fate of atropine and hyoscine
Both atropine and hyoscine are readily absorbed from the intestine after oral administration and they are almost completely absorbed into the bloodstream within 2 hours. Both substances are considerably bound to plasma proteins and their elimination by the kidneys is usually complete within 24 hours. About 50 per cent of an oral dose of either substance appears unchanged in the urine with the majority of the remainder being present in the form of metabolites. These drugs are slowly absorbed from mucous membranes and there may be some slight systemic absorption from preparations applied to the intact skin.

Clinical uses of atropine and hyoscine
Both substances find widespread clinical usage and are present in many preparations intended for internal use and in a few preparations intended for external application. The major

clinical uses for these drugs are dependent on their effects on the heart, gastrointestinal tract, brain and eyes.

Heart

Atropine or hyoscine is commonly administered as part of premedication before general anaesthesia. Their use for this purpose is based firstly on their effect in preventing excessive vagal slowing of the heart and thus reducing the risk of cardiac arrest and, secondly, on their action in reducing the secretion of saliva and of bronchial mucus. This latter effect is of particular importance when ether is used as an anaesthetic agent since it stimulates the secretions of the salivary and bronchial glands. Hyoscine is usually preferred to atropine as a premedicant since it has sedative properties which help to calm the patient. However, both atropine and hyoscine may, rarely and unpredictably, cause marked excitement even in low doses. Atropine and hyoscine are each effective in the treatment of vagal syncope, a condition caused by an overly-active carotid sinus reflex leading to excessive vagal slowing of the heart and fainting.

Atropine is sometimes used to treat irregularities of the heartbeat caused by partial block of the conducting tissues and also to abolish the profound bradycardia which, in some patients, follows myocardial infarction.

Gastrointestinal tract

Preparations containing solanaceous alkaloids are widely used in the treatment of disorders of the gastrointestinal tract including gastric and duodenal ulceration. Their usefulness in these conditions probably depends mainly on their spasmolytic effect in relaxing smooth muscle which in turn is probably only partly dependent on their antimuscarinic effects. Atropine-like drugs are relatively ineffective in reducing gastric acid secretion and their spasmolytic effects are variable and to some extent depend on the existing tone and motility of the gastrointestinal tract. Atropine is of value in the treatment of spasm of the pylorus and of the bile ducts.

Brain

Both atropine and hyoscine are effective in treating the rigidity of Parkinson's disease (*paralysis agitans*). It is probable that this effect is due to antagonism of acetylcholine actions in the brain. These alkaloids, and extracts of plants containing them, have, to a large extent, been replaced in the treatment of this condition by the newer synthetic antimuscarinics, such as benzhexol, which are reputed to have fewer peripheral side-effects. Hyoscine has well-marked sedative effects and has been used to treat manic states such as those occurring as a result of alcoholism and during withdrawal of drugs of dependence. Hyoscine, often in combination with pethidine, is used in obstetrics to produce a relaxed state of the patient called 'twilight sleep' which is associated with amnesia and partial analgesia. Both atropine and hyoscine are effective in preventing motion sickness and, to a lesser extent, in treating it once begun. This action is believed to be central in origin and in practice hyoscine is usually preferred to atropine presumably on the basis that its ratio of central to peripheral actions is believed to be greater than that of atropine.

The eyes

Solutions of atropine and occasionally of hyoscine are instilled onto the surface of the eyes to produce mydriasis and cycloplegia during examinations of the eyes for refractive errors. When used for this purpose both drugs produce effects lasting several days or more and nowadays a semi-synthetic antimuscarinic, homatropine, is usually used because of its prompt onset and relatively brief duration of action. However, the persistent effects of hyoscine and atropine are sometimes utilised in the treatment of inflammation of the iris (*iritis*) since the prolonged immobilisation of the ciliary muscle and iris which they cause help to prevent the formation of adhesions. The ophthalmic use of atropine and hyoscine, especially in the elderly, carries a greater risk of provoking a dangerous increase of intraocular pressure than does the use of homatropine. Anticholinesterases are the logical antidotes to the effects of these drugs on the eye as in other tissues.

Miscellaneous uses of atropine and hyoscine

A number of uses for these drugs are probably more dependent on their spasmolytic effects on smooth muscle than on their specific antimuscarinic activity. Thus they have been used to treat spasm of the smooth muscle in the respiratory tract in bronchial asthma and whooping cough, the ureters in ureteral spasm, the uterus in painful menstruation (*dysmenorrhoea*) and bladder in urinary incontinence (*enuresis*). A combination of atropine and adrenaline in the form of a spray solution for inhalation was formerly much used to relieve excessive bronchoconstriction in asthma but has now been largely superseded by specific and orally effective sympathomimetics (Chapter 9).

Extracts of solanaceous plants were at one time used in preparations for external application to the skin and mucous membranes to ease the pain occurring in conditions such as lumbago, sciatica and haemorrhoids. It is not clear which property (if any) of these substances is responsible for these uses. It is possible that local anaesthesia may play some part in easing the pain of haemorrhoids and it has been suggested that these substances may act as counter-irritants to ease muscular pains. However, there is no clear evidence that these preparations are effective in these conditions but their use persists and preparations such as Belladonna Liniment are still used and receive official (BPC) recognition.

Small doses of atropine, hyoscine or some related antimuscarinic are present in some 'cold-cure' remedies. Their usefulness in such preparations is based on their ability to dry up nasal and possibly bronchial secretions and thus to increase the comfort of the sufferer without altering the course of the infection. Atropine or hyoscine may be used to treat excessive sweating (hyperhidrosis).

Preparations and doses of atropine and hyoscine

Atropine is usually administered in the form of Atropine Sulphate BP either as tablets (usual strength 0·5 mg) or as the official (BP, BNF) injection (containing 0·4, 0·6, 0·8 or 1 mg in one ml). The usual adult dose of atropine sulphate is 0·25 to 2 mg although up to 4 mg of tablets and 3 mg of injection may be given in any 24 hour period. For ophthalmic use atropine is available as an eye ointment (BP, BNF) containing 1 per cent and as eye drops (BPC, BNF) containing 0·5 or 1 per cent of atropine sulphate.

Hyoscine is usually administered systemically as the hydrobromide in adult doses of 300 to 600 micrograms. The official (BP, BNF) tablets each contain 300 micrograms and the injection (BP) 400 micrograms in one ml. For ophthalmic use the BP eye ointment contains 0·25 per cent and the BP eye drops 0·5 per cent of hyoscine hydrobromide.

In addition to the pure alkaloids, crude extracts of solanaceous plants are still used in considerable quantities and receive official recognition. Thus, extracts of Belladonna Herb BP are used in many liquid and tablet preparations for the treatment of digestive and intestinal symptoms. These preparations often contain antacids and sometimes additionally small doses of barbiturates. Extracts of Belladonna Root BPC are used mainly in preparations intended for external use such as Belladonna Liniment BPC. Extracts of Hyoscyamus, particularly the tincture (BP) are used for their antispasmodic effects on the intestine and ureters, whilst Tincture of Strammonium BP is used to relieve bronchoconstriction and to treat Parkinson's Disease.

Atropine, hyoscine and extracts of solanaceous plants are constituents of a very large number of proprietary medicines recommended by the makers for a wide variety of clinical conditions. In general, the advantages of many of these preparations over the usually much less expensive official preparations resides in their often greater pharmaceutical elegance and hence patient acceptability rather than increased clinical efficacy.

Synthetic antimuscarinic agents
A great deal of pharmacological and chemical endeavour on the part of the pharmaceutical industry has gone into the production of numerous synthetic compounds possessing muscarinic receptor blocking activity. The object of this endeavour has been to produce compounds with similar blocking activity to atropine but with actions restricted to certain organs. Thus in the treatment of Parkinson's disease only central antimuscarinic effects are required, the peripheral effects on heart, eye and gastrointestinal tract being, in this instance, unwanted side-effects. Conversely, drugs designed for their effects on the gastrointestinal tract are not required to produce effects on the brain or eye. The two main clinical conditions in which antimuscarinics have been shown to be useful are Parkinson's disease and ulceration of the stomach and/or small intestine in which latter conditions they reduce gastric acid secretion and motility of the gastrointestinal tract. A less important use for synthetic antimuscarinics is in ophthalmology to produce mydriasis and cycloplegia mainly to aid examination of the eye for refractive errors. For ophthalmic use the aim is to produce antimuscarinics with a rapid onset and much shorter duration of action than the solanaceous alkaloids.

The present status of antimuscarinic substances in the treatment of Parkinson's disease is in some doubt since the discovery of the beneficial effects of the amino-acid L-DOPA in the treatment of this condition. However, many antimuscarinics have been marketed for their anti-Parkinsonian effects and several, of which benzhexol (ARTANE) is an example, are still widely used. These compounds are beyond the scope of this monograph and will not be described further except to mention that it is doubtful whether they are significantly more selective for central actions than the solanaceous alkaloids when used in equi-effective doses.

More than 50 synthetic antimuscarinics have been tried clinically for their effects on the gastrointestinal tract in the treatment of ulceration of the stomach and duodenum and some 20 or so are still commercially available in the United Kingdom. The number of drugs and preparations available clearly indicates both the lack of clear-cut superiority of any one agent over the others and also the need for a really effective remedy for the treatment of gastrointestinal disturbances. The major problem in using antimuscarinics to reduce motility and secretion of the gastrointestinal tract is that both effects are relatively resistant to parasympathetic blockade and effective doses produce many unwanted effects in other tissues. Recently, substances have been described which specifically block receptors (H_2 receptors) on which histamine acts to promote gastric acid secretion. These substances, one of which cimetidine (TAGAMET) is commercially available, produce in man a marked and long-lasting decrease in gastric acid secretion and are said to be effective in the treatment of ulceration of the gastrointestinal tract. The clinical status of these compounds has yet to be established but they would seem to hold more promise of future useful clinical development than do the antimuscarinics.

The synthetic antimuscarinics may be divided into two main classes; those structurally related to atropine and a much larger group of substances most of which bear little structural resemblance to atropine. In both groups the main chemical modification which has been made of the proposed active sites for atropine-like activity is quaternisation of the nitrogen atom. The quaternary compounds are considerably ionised at bodily pH, are less well absorbed after oral administration than the tertiary compounds, possess some degree of autonomic ganglion blocking activity and do not penetrate into the central nervous system to any extent and therefore do not produce the central effects of the solanaceous alkaloids. It is likely that the ganglion blocking activity of these compounds contributes to their effects in reducing gastric acid secretion and gastrointestinal motility. In addition, many of these compounds possess direct smooth muscle relaxant properties which contribute to their useful antispasmodic effects and which is probably more related to

their local anaesthetic effects rather than to their specific muscarinic receptor blocking actions. Atropine and other solanaceous
alkaloids likewise possess local anaesthetic activity and part of
their useful antispasmodic effects are probably due to direct
relaxant effects on smooth muscle.

Antimuscarinics structurally-related to atropine

Homatropine Hydrobromide BP

$$H_2C-CH———CH_2 \quad \quad OH$$
$$| \quad \quad | \quad \quad |$$
$$N-CH_3 \quad CH-O-CO-CH-\langle \bigcirc \rangle \quad \cdot \overline{H}Br$$
$$| \quad \quad |$$
$$H_2C-CH———CH_2$$

This substance, which was the first synthetic atropine-like drug
produced, is used almost exclusively in ophthalmology as a
mydriatic and cycloplegic and to treat corneal ulceration and
iritis. The great advantage of homatropine over atropine or
hyoscine is that its cycloplegic effect is briefer, normal accommodation usually returning within 24 hours of use compared with
up to a week or more with the solanaceous alkaloids. Homatropine has found occasional oral use for its anti-secretory and
relaxant effects on the gastrointestinal tract.

Clinical uses and dosage. For internal use the adult dose is
0·5 to 2 mg. The official (BPC, BNF) eye drops contain 1 or
2 per cent Homatropine Hydrobromide BP. In common with
the other solanaceous alkaloids homatropine may cause irritation
of the cornea in some sensitive persons. The quaternary derivative homatropine methobromide is sometimes used orally in
adult doses up to 20 mg per day to treat gastrointestinal symptoms and also spasm of the bile duct, urinary bladder or ureters.
It is present with phenobarbitone in the proprietary preparation
PEPTACOL.

Atropine Methonitrate BP

$$H_2C———CH———CH_2 \quad \quad CH_2OH$$
$$| \quad \quad |+ \quad \quad | \quad \quad |$$
$$H_3C-N-CH_3 \quad CH-O-CO-CH-\langle \bigcirc \rangle \quad \cdot \overline{N}O_3$$
$$| \quad \quad |$$
$$H_2C———CH———CH_2$$

This quaternary derivative of atropine has both potent antimuscarinic and ganglion blocking activities. It lacks the central
effects of atropine.

Clinical uses and dosage. The main use of this substance is in the treatment of congenital hypertrophic stenosis and pyloric spasm of infants when it is used in doses of 200 to 600 micrograms. For this use it is available commercially as a 0·6 per cent solution in 90 per cent ethanol for oral use (EUMYDRIN DROPS).

Atropine methonitrate is also an ingredient of Compound Adrenaline and Atropine Spray BPC which finds occasional use in the treatment of asthma. Atropine methonitrate and the closely-related atropine methobromide have each been used for their local effects on the eye. They have a shorter duration of action as mydriatics than atropine but offer no advantage over homatropine.

Hyoscine Methobromide

This substance has both antimuscarinic and ganglion blocking activity. It lacks the central effects of hyoscine, is less well absorbed by mouth but has an anti-secretory and antispasmodic effect on the gastrointestinal tract lasting about 8 hours.

Clinical uses and dosage. Hyoscine methobromide is mainly used for its effects on the gastrointestinal tract and is used in oral adult doses of up to 20 mg per day. It is marketed as tablets each containing 2·5 mg active ingredient under the trade-name of PAMINE.

The closely-related substance hyoscine butylbromide has been widely used for its effects on the gut and for treating spasm of bile ducts, ureters and uterus. It is less well absorbed by mouth than the methobromide and is used in oral doses of up to 100 mg daily or more effectively by intramuscular or intravenous injection in doses up to 60 mg daily. The trade name is BUSCO-PAN.

Synthetic antimuscarinics not closely related structurally to atropine

This group includes a large number of substances some of which are used exclusively in the treatment of Parkinson's disease. These latter substances will not be described and the present account will be restricted to a selection of substances which are used clinically for the peripheral effects on the autonomic nerves usually of the gastrointestinal tract and eye. Detailed information is given only on those substances which have received official (BP, BPC or BNF) recognition or are widely used in clinical practice. The approved names, clinical uses, doses and trade names of most of the other compounds available in the United Kingdom are given in Table 6.1.

Table 6.1 Synthetic antimuscarinic drugs used clinically for their peripheral (systemic) effects.

Antimuscarinic	Trade name	Major clinical uses
Clidinium bromide	LIBRAXIN (chlordiazepoxide also present)	Peptic ulceration, dyspepsia, irritable colon.
Emepronium bromide	CETIPRIN	Urinary frequency and incontinence.
Glycopyrronium bromide	ROBINUL	Peptic ulceration
Isopropamide iodide	TYRIMIDE	Gastrointestinal disturbances
Mepenzolate bromide	CANTIL	Spasm or hypermotility of the gastrointestinal tract
Penthienate methobromide	MONODRAL	Peptic ulceration and gastric hypermotility
Pipenzolate bromide	PIPTAL	Peptic ulceration
Piperidolate hydrochloride	DACTIL	Gastrointestinal spasm

Oxyphenonium Bromide

Oxyphenonium is a quaternary compound with marked antimuscarinic and ganglion blocking activity. Large doses may block nicotinic acetylcholine receptors in voluntary muscle and give rise to muscular weakness.

Clinical uses and dosage. Its main use is in the treatment of gastrointestinal ulceration where it is used in oral adult doses of up to 40 mg per day. It finds some use as a premedicant and in ophthalmology as a substitute for solanaceous alkaloids in persons intolerant to them. The trade name is ANTRENYL.

Oxyphencyclimine Hydrochloride BP

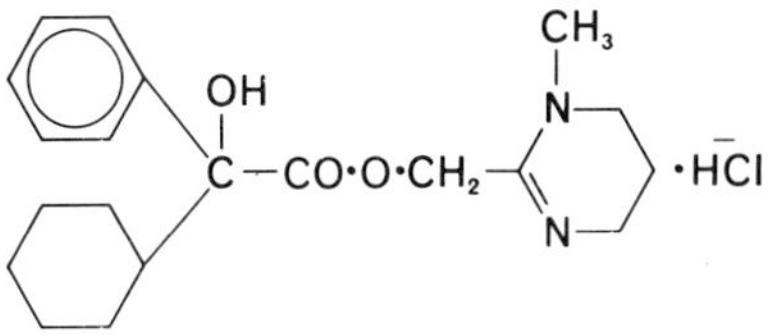

This substance is similar structurally to oxyphenonium except that it is not a quaternary compound and therefore is virtually without ganglion blocking activity. However, it has direct smooth muscle relaxant properties and a longer duration of action than oxphenonium.

Clinical uses and dosage. It is mainly used for its effects on the gastrointestinal tract in adult doses of 15–20 mg per day. The official (BP) tablets each contain 5 mg of active substance and it is also available in the same form under the trade-name of DARICON.

Poldine Methylsulphate BP

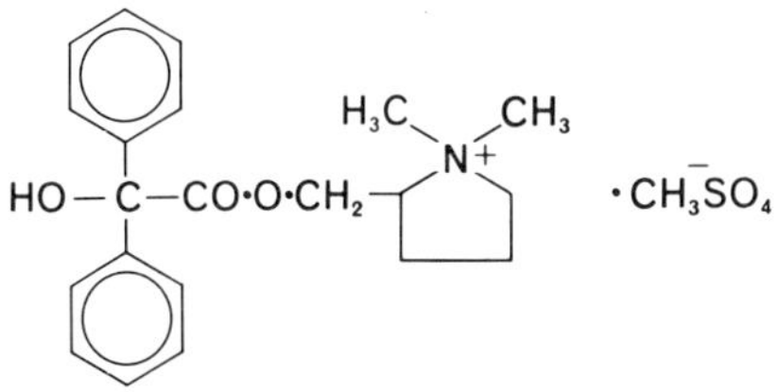

This quaternary substance has both antimuscarinic and ganglion blocking activity.

Clinical uses and dosage. It is used mostly for its effects on the gastrointestinal tract. The adult dose is 10–30 mg orally per day; the tablets of the BP each contain 2 mg. It is also available under the trade name NACTON.

Propantheline Bromide BP

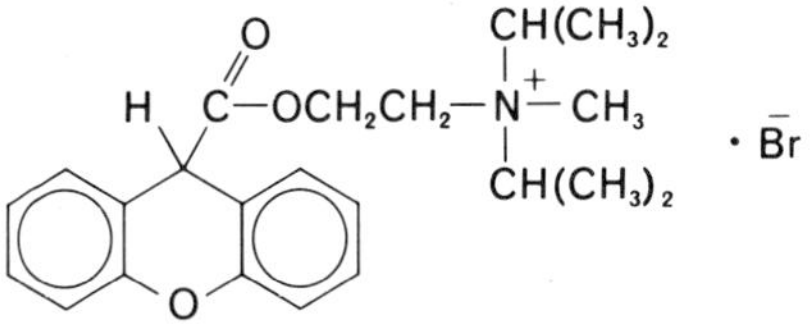

This quaternary substance has been widely used clinically; it has antimuscarinic and ganglion blocking activity. High doses may cause muscular weakness due to blockade of acetylcholine (nicotinic) receptors in voluntary muscle.

Clinical uses and dosage. It is used for its effects in depressing gastric acid secretion and gastrointestinal motility. The official (BP, BNF) tablets each contain 15 mg propantheline and the adult dose is up to 45 mg per day. The trade name is PRO-BANTHINE.

Dicyclomine Hydrochloride BP

This tertiary amine has relatively weak antimuscarinic potency and owes most of its antispasmodic action to its high local anaesthetic potency. It has only a slight effect in reducing secretion of gastric acid.

Clinical uses and dosage. Dicyclomine is used mainly for its effects in reducing gastrointestinal spasm resulting from gastric or duodenal ulceration. The oral adult dose is 30 to 60 mg per day and it is officially available as 10 mg tablets (BP, BNF) and as an elixir containing 10 mg per 5 ml (BNF). It is available under the trade name of MERBENTYL and is also combined with antacids in several other proprietary preparations.

Synthetic antimuscarinics used in ophthalmology

Cyclopentolate Hydrochloride BP

This substance has the same uses and similar duration as homatropine. It is used in patients in whom solanaceous alkaloids cause corneal irritation. It is used as 0·5 or 1 per cent solutions and is commercially available (MYDRILATE).

Lachesine Chloride BPC

$$HO-\underset{\underset{\bigcirc}{\overset{\bigcirc}{|}}}{C}-CO \cdot O \cdot CH_2CH_2 - \underset{\underset{CH_3}{|}}{\overset{\overset{CH_3}{|}}{N^+}} - C_2H_5 \cdot \bar{C}l$$

This quaternary compound has actions on the eye midway between those of atropine and homatropine; the maximum effect on the pupil and accommodation occurs within one hour and begins to subside after 5 to 6 hours. The official (BPC) eye drops contain 1 per cent lachesine chloride.

Tropicamide

$$\text{\Large\textcircled{}} - CH - \underset{\overset{\|}{O}}{C} - \underset{}{N} - CH_2 - \text{\Large\textcircled{}N}$$

with substituents CH_2OH and C_2H_5

This compound is a very short-acting mydriatic and cycloplegic. A 1 per cent solution produces a maximum effect within 20 minutes of instillation into the eye and persisting for about 20 minutes; full recovery of accommodation occurs within 6 hours. It is widely used for examination of the eyes for refractive errors. A 0·5 per cent solution produces mydriasis without cycloplegia. The eye drops (BNF) contain 0·5 or 1 per cent tropicamide and it is also available under the trade name of MYDRIACYL.

SUMMARY

Atropine is the classical competitive antagonist for the muscarinic effects of acetylcholine in the body. Atropine and the closely related substance, hyoscine, are alkaloids present in several plants of the solanaceae family. Atropine and hyoscine are potent and specific antagonists for muscarinic receptors. However, in some tissues, such as the urinary bladder and gastrointestinal tract, they are more effective in abolishing the effects of parasympathomimetic substances exogenously administered than they are against acetylcholine released from parasympathetic nerve endings. The major clinical uses of atropine and hyoscine are based on their effects in blocking muscarinic receptors in the heart, eye, gastrointestinal tract and brain. These drugs prevent excessive vagal slowing of the heart, are potent and long-acting mydriatics, inhibit tone, motility and secretion of the gastrointestinal tract and are useful in the treatment of Parkinson's disease and motion sickness. The solanaceous alkaloids have a number of other uses including reduction of secretion of sweat, saliva and bronchial mucus and by external application to ease pain in various muscular and inflammatory conditions.

Several synthetic compounds related to atropine and hyoscine have been prepared with the object of producing drugs with a more selective action and/or briefer duration. Homatropine is one such compound which is widely used in ophthalmology because of its short duration of action compared with atropine and hyoscine. Quaternisation of the nitrogen atom of hyoscine and atropine produces substances which have autonomic ganglion blocking actions in addition to antimuscarinic effects. These compounds produce a more marked effect on the gastro-intestinal tract than on many other tissues.

A large number of synthetic compounds with antimuscarinic actions, but bearing little chemical resemblance to atropine, have been prepared and tried clinically. Some of these compounds are quaternised and have ganglion blocking as well as antimuscarinic effects and some possess additional non-specific relaxant effects on smooth muscle. Some of the non-quaternary compounds, such as benzhexol, penetrate into the brain and have been used to treat Parkinson's disease. The quaternary compounds such as oxyphenonium and propantheline do not penetrate readily into the brain and are used mainly for their effects in reducing tone, motility and secretion of the gastrointestinal tract in patients suffering from gastric or peptic ulceration. The amount of selectivity obtained with synthetic antimuscarinic compounds is relatively small and few of the compounds are significantly more useful clinically than the solanaceous alkaloids when used in equi-effective dosage.

REFERENCES

Bezold, A. von & Bloebaum, F. (1867) Ueber die physiologischen wirkungen des schwefelsauren atropins. *Untersuch. physiol. Lab. Würzburg.*, **1**, 1–72.
Dale, H. H. (1914) The action of certain esters and ethers of choline, and their relation to muscarine. *J. Pharmac. exp. Ther.*, **2**, 147–190.
Mein, (1833) Ueber die darstellung des atropins in weissen krystallen. *Liebigs. Ann.* **6**, 67–72.

GENERAL READING

Ambache, N. (1955) The use and limitations of atropine for pharmacological studies of autonomic effectors. *Pharmac. Revs.*, **7**, 467–494.

Barlow, R. B. (1964) *Introduction to Chemical Pharmacology*, London: Menthuen & Co. Ltd.

Bowman, W. C., Rand, M. J. & West, G. B. (1968) *Textbook of Pharmacology*, Oxford:Blackwell Scientific Publications.

Brimblecombe, R. W. (1974) *Drug Actions on Cholinergic Systems*, London: The Macmillan Press Ltd.

Innes, I. R. & Nickerson, M. (1975) Atropine, scopolamine, and related antimuscarinic drugs. In *The Pharmacological Basis of Therapeutics*, 5th edn., pp 514–532, (eds.) Goodman, L. S. & Gilman, A. New York, Macmillan Publishing Co.

Martindale, (1977) *The Extra Pharmacopoeia*, 27th edn., London: The Pharmaceutical Press.

7

Drugs acting at autonomic ganglia; ganglion stimulants and ganglion blockers

The events occurring when nerve impulses traverse the synapse between pre and postganglionic autonomic nerves were outlined in Chapter 3. Acetylcholine is released from the preganglionic nerve terminals and combines with receptors situated on the cell bodies of postganglionic neurones causing depolarisation of the cell membrane and propagation of action potentials (excitatory postsynaptic potentials) in the postganglionic nerve fibres. The acetylcholine receptors on autonomic ganglia and on the cells of the adrenal medullae are predominantly of the nicotinic type being stimulated by low and blocked by high concentrations of nicotine. Recent studies suggest that the transmission process across autonomic ganglia, especially of the sympathetic system, may be more complicated in its finest detail and may involve neurotransmitters in addition to acetylcholine and receptor types other than nicotinic. However, the simple pathway outlined above is generally considered to be the primary transmission process and adequately explains the major pharmacological effects produced by commonly used stimulants and blockers of autonomic ganglia. Some details of recent experimental work on ganglionic transmission will be given towards the end of the present chapter.

Autonomic ganglion stimulants

Nicotine

Nicotine is the colourless, volatile and highly toxic liquid alkaloid obtained from the leaves of the tobacco plant *Nicotiana tabacum*. It is a strongly basic substance, readily soluble in water, and forms neutral water-soluble salts. Despite having no therapeutic uses it is nevertheless one of the world's most widely used drugs and experimentally it has been extensively studied for more than a century.

The actions of nicotine at autonomic ganglia were first examined in detail by Langley & Dickinson (1889) who used the superior cervical sympathetic ganglion of the anaesthetised cat. This ganglion has been widely utilised in studies involving the autonomic ganglionic transmission process since it is accessible and can be prepared to allow of electrical stimulation of its pre and/or postganglionic fibres. Structures innervated by post-ganglionic fibres arising from the superior cervical ganglion include the radial muscle of the iris and the smooth muscle of the third eye-lid (*the nictitating membrane*) both of which produce reproducible and measurable responses when their sympathetic nerves are stimulated. Langley & Dickinson administered nicotine by painting a 1 per cent aqueous solution of it directly onto the ganglion and found that it initially stimulated the ganglion and subsequently blocked transmission through it. The mechanism of the ganglion blockade produced by nicotine is not entirely clear. Initially, it seemed likely that it was causing blockade by persistent depolarisation of the postsynaptic mem-brane thus densitising it to the depolarising action of acetyl-choline released from preganglionic nerve endings. It is known that acetylcholine itself can produce this type of block if ad-ministered in large doses or after inhibition of acetylcholinest-erase. More recent work suggests that nicotine behaves as a partial agonist at the ganglion producing initial depolarisation which subsides despite the continued attachment of nicotine to the receptors; after the initial stimulant action nicotine probably blocks conduction through the ganglion by competition with acetylcholine for nicotinic receptors. A similar type of blockade may occur at the neuro-effector junction in voluntary muscle with muscle relaxant drugs of the depolarising type such as succinylcholine and has been called 'dual mode of action block'.

General pharmacological effects of nicotine

Nicotine produces a variety of effects in the body many of which oppose each other and are therefore difficult to analyse. It stimulates and then blocks both sympathetic and parasym-pathetic ganglia and also the chromaffin cells of the adrenal medullae. It also stimulates and may block the neuro-effector junctions in voluntary muscle, some sensory nerve endings, sympathetic nerve endings and at multiple sites within the central nervous system. Analysis of the actions of nicotine in the body is further complicated by the fact that its spectrum of activity is largely dependent on the dose administered. It is not surprising that such a drug finds no clinical use and the reasons for its use as a drug of pleasure, apparently enjoyed, by many millions of persons remains an intriguing mystery. It is not clear which of the many effects of nicotine are prized by smokers although actions within the central nervous system seem to be most important. Tobacco contains a number of substances other than nicotine and even more are formed when it is slowly burned; however, all the evidence suggests that it is nicotine itself which endows tobacco smoking with its pleasurable qualities. The damage to health caused by tobacco smoking has been well publicised and each year it is responsible for many avoidable deaths from carcinoma of the lung, bronchitis and cardiovascular disease with all of which conditions it has been implicated. It is to be hoped that in the future increasing efforts in health education, particularly those directed at the young, will help to reduce this death toll.

Tetramethylammonium salts (TMA)

$$H_3C - \overset{\overset{\textstyle CH_3}{|}}{\underset{\underset{\textstyle CH_3}{|}}{\overset{+}{N}}} - CH_3 \cdot \bar{C}l$$

tetramethylammonium chloride

The tetramethylammonium ion (TMA) was shown by Marshall (1913) and by Burn & Dale (1915) to produce similar actions to nicotine at autonomic ganglia, the adrenal medullae and the neuro-effector junction of voluntary muscle. It is of similar potency to nicotine in its ganglion stimulant effects but is weaker than nicotine in producing ganglion blockade. Thus it is possible to administer repeated doses of TMA and obtain reproducible ganglion stimulant effects. Drugs such as nicotine which tend to rapidly lose their effectiveness on repeated administration are said to exhibit *tachyphylaxis*. TMA is therefore less tachyphylactic than nicotine and for this reason is often preferred to it in experimental studies in which a reproducible ganglion stimulant effect is desired. TMA is therefore a useful experimental tool but has no clinical uses.

DMPP (1, 1-dimethyl-4-phenylpiperazinium iodide)

DMPP iodide

This substance is a very potent nicotinic agonist which like TMA has stronger agonist than antagonist activity and has been used in experimental studies involving ganglionic transmission. DMPP has also been shown to possess the property of preventing the release of noradrenaline from sympathetic nerve endings in response to postganglionic stimulation, although this action does not appear to be related to either stimulation or blockade of nicotinic receptors.

Ganglion blocking agents

Drugs such as nicotine and TMA which markedly stimulate the nicotinic receptors in autonomic ganglia and the adrenal medullae are of experimental interest but have no clinical applications. However, drugs which compete with acetylcholine for the same receptors without causing initial stimulation may be used clinically to treat sustained elevated arterial blood pressure (*hypertension*). The ganglion blockers are now little used in the treatment of this condition but their introduction into therapy in the early 1950's heralded the beginning of a new era of effective therapy for this common and life-shortening condition. The autonomic ganglion blockers are therefore of considerable historical interest, are widely used experimentally, and have a small but not insignificant place in therapy.

Tetraethylammonium salts (TEA)

tetraethylammonium chloride

Tetraethylammonium ion (TEA) is structurally the simplest of the ganglion blockers and was the first synthetic substance with this type of action to be tested experimentally (Marshall, 1913; Burn & Dale, 1915). Following these initial reports the drug was virtually ignored for 30 years until interest in its actions were revived by Acheson and his colleagues (Acheson & Moe, 1946;

Acheson & Pereira, 1946). It was subsequently tested in man and was found to lower blood pressure in hypertensive patients. However, it is poorly absorbed by mouth and has a very short duration of action making it unsuitable for routine clinical use.

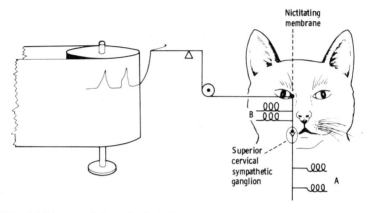

Fig. 7.1 Diagram of the cat's nictitating membrane preparation. The membrane, which is composed of smooth muscle and cartilage is attached to a thread which is passed over a pulley to a lever writing on a revolving drum. The sympathetic innervation of the membrane may be electrically stimulated via electrodes placed either preganglionically (A) or postganglionically (B) to produce contractions of the membrane. It is more usual at present to record muscle contractions in this and other preparations by means of an electronic transducer the output of which may be amplified and recorded using an electronic recorder.

Hexamethonium

$$H_3C-\underset{\underset{CH_3}{|}}{\overset{\overset{CH_3}{|}}{N^+}}-(CH_2)_6-\underset{\underset{CH_3}{|}}{\overset{\overset{CH_3}{|}}{N^+}}-CH_3 \cdot \bar{Br}$$

hexamethonium bromide

This substance was the first ganglion blocker to be widely used in man and also one of the first effective drugs for the treatment of hypertension. Hexamethonium was one of a series of poly-methylene bistrimethylammonium compounds described and tested in animals independently by Paton & Zaimis (1949) and by Barlow & Ing (1948). These compounds are symetrical molecules composed of two quaternary nitrogen groups separated by a chain of methylene (CH_2) groups of variable length. It was found that autonomic ganglion blocking activity in this series reached a peak when the methylene bridge consisted of six carbon atoms (hexamethonium). This compound is often called 'C$_6$' by experimenters. Increase in the length of the methylene chain above six carbon atoms led to a sharp drop in ganglion blocking activity and to the eventual appearance of skeletal muscle paralysing activity of the depolarising type which reached a peak with compound C$_{10}$ (decamethonium).

Hexamethonium, like TEA, produces ganglion blockade without initial stimulation but it is more potent and has a longer

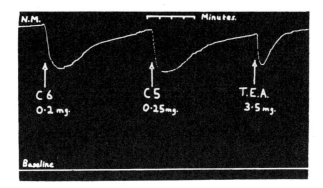

Fig. 7.2 Comparison of the effectiveness of ganglion blocking drugs on the nictitating membrane of a chloralose-anaesthetised cat. The preganglionic fibres of the superior cervical sympathetic nerve supplying the nictitating membrane were stimulated electrically at a rate of 10 impulses per second throughout the experiment to keep the membrane under a constant degree of tension. At the arrows ganglion blocking drugs were injected intravenously and produced a temporary reduction in impulse flow through the ganglion. 0·2 mg of hexamethonium (C$_6$) produced a similar degree of blockade as 0·25 mg of pentamethonium (C$_5$) but tetraethylammonium ion (TEA) produced only a small and transient blocking effect at a dose of 3·5 mg. (From Paton & Zaimis 1949).

duration of action than TEA. In common with the other drugs of this class hexamethonium has been often tested on the superior cervical ganglion of the cat (see Figs. 7.1 and 7.2). Both hexamethonium and TEA are specific for the nicotinic receptors in autonomic ganglia and adrenal medullae and neither produce significant blockade of the acetylcholine receptors in voluntary muscle in doses up to a hundred times greater than those needed to block ganglionic transmission. This fact, taken together with the far greater effect of decamethonium at somatic nerve muscle junctions than at ganglionic synapses, is further evidence of the marked differences between the acetylcholine receptors at the two sites.

Cardiovascular effects of hexamethonium

The cardiovascular effects of hexamethonium have been well studied but all the ganglion blocking substances produce qualitatively similar effects on this system in man. Ganglion blockade reduces arterial blood pressure by preventing the passage of nerve impulses across sympathetic ganglia thus abolishing vasoconstrictor tone and producing a relaxation of the smooth muscle in the walls of the blood vessels. The fall in blood pressure produced is therefore largely as a result of reduced peripheral resistance due to vasodilatation of systemic blood vessels, particularly the arterioles, which contribute to the peripheral resistance. These drugs have a more variable effect on the cardiac output but generally lower it because of reduced venous return to the heart resulting from pooling of blood in dilated veins. In patients with cardiac failure the fall in blood pressure caused by ganglion blockade may allow of more complete cardiac emptying with a consequent increase in cardiac output. The effect of hexamethonium and related drugs on heart rate is variable and depends on the initial level of vagal tone. If the initial rate is high then ganglion blockade may lower it but the more usual effects of full doses is a slight tachycardia.

Since the fall in blood pressure produced by these drugs is dependent on the number of impulses travelling in the vaso-constrictor nerves it follows that the drugs are more effective if the patient is standing, when sympathetic outflow is high, than when lying when sympathetic activity is low (see Fig. 7.3). Because of their dependence on posture ganglion blockers are said to produce an *orthostatic* fall in blood pressure. In addition to blocking the resting tone in vasoconstrictor nerves, ganglion blockers also abolish the increases in neural activity which occur during the sympathetic cardiovascular reflexes involved in postural changes of the body. Thus when a person stands up from a lying position there is an initial sharp fall in blood pressure due to pooling of blood in the legs under the influence of gravity and a consequent reduction in venous return and cardiac output. The fall in blood pressure is detected by pressure-sensitive (*baroreceptors*) present in the carotid sinus and aortic arch which, via neural connections with blood pressure-regulating centres in the hind-brain, bring about a rapid increase in sympathetic drive to the blood vessels resulting in vasoconstriction and a return of the blood pressure to its former level. Following ganglion blockade the reflex vasoconstriction is abolished and, on standing, the blood pressure may fall to a very low level (*postural hypotension*) which often produces fainting due to cerebral ischaemia. This unwanted effect on cardiovascular reflex mechanisms is also produced by some other drugs which are used to treat hypertension (*antihypertensive agents*) and is often very troublesome to the patient.

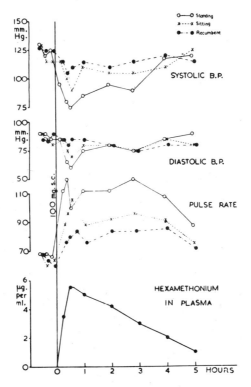

Fig. 7.3 Effect of hexamethonium (100 mg subcutaneously at time 0) on the systolic and diastolic blood pressures and pulse rate of a normal subject in standing, sitting and recumbent postures. The lower record shows the plasma level of hexamethonium at various times after the injection. (From Morrison & Paton, 1953).

Unwanted effects of hexamethonium

Hexamethonium, like the other drugs in this class, blocks transmission equally effectively in parasympathetic as in sympathetic ganglia and this leads to a number of unwanted effects some of which seriously disrupt the patient's life. The effects of autonomic ganglion blockade are predictable from a knowledge of the distribution and functions of autonomic fibres to various tissues. The unwanted effects of hexamethonium are on peripheral smooth muscle-containing tissues since the quaternary substances do not penetrate into the central nervous system. However, some of the later non-quaternary compounds also produce unwanted effects on the brain.

The eye

The overall effect of ganglion blockade is an incomplete mydriasis as a result of blockade of sympathetic and parasympathetic nerves to the iris. In addition, the effectiveness of the parasympathetic supply to the ciliary muscle is reduced leading to partial paralysis of accommodation. The patient may therefore suffer from blurred vision and difficulty in focusing.

Glandular secretions

Ganglion blockers reduce the secretion of digestive juices from the stomach and small intestine by blocking the parasympathetic ganglia. Secretion of saliva and sweat is also decreased. Patients may therefore complain of digestive problems and dry mouth.

Gastrointestinal tract

The tone and motility of all parts of the gastrointestinal tract are reduced by blockade of the parasympathetic ganglia in the myenteric (Auerbach's) plexus. This results in a slowing of gastric emptying after meals and often to severe constipation due to reduced tone and motility of the large bowel. Full doses of ganglion blockers carry the risk of a complete blockage of intestinal motility (*paralytic ileus*) which is sometimes fatal.

Urinary bladder

Blockade of the parasympathetic ganglia of the pelvic parasympathetic nerves produces difficulty in complete emptying of the bladder and may sometimes lead to serious urinary retention.

Sex organs

Ganglion blockade produces serious consequences to sexual performance in the male often producing complete impotence. Erection is prevented by blockade of the parasympathetic fibres of the nervi erigentes and ejaculation by abolition of sympathetic transmission to the vasa deferentia, seminal ducts and seminal vesicles.

Absorption and uses of hexamethonium

Hexamethonium is poorly and erratically absorbed when given by mouth; only 10–15 per cent of an oral dose finding its way into the bloodstream. The most reliable method of lowering blood pressure with the drug is by subcutaneous or intramuscular injection. When used over long periods to treat hypertension it was found that tolerance to the antihypertensive effect of hexamethonium often developed. The mechanism of this tolerance is not fully understood but is believed to be at least partly due to the supersensitivity of vascular smooth muscle to the vasoconstrictor action of noradrenaline which is induced by hexamethonium. Hexamethonium is now rarely used to treat chronic hypertension but it finds occasional use to produce controlled hypotension during surgery in order to reduce bleeding. In this technique the drug is administered intravenously and the level of arterial pressure can be controlled by adjusting the rate of infusion of the blocker and/or the degree of tilt of the patient. This technique (*'bloodless field' surgery*) is of particular value in plastic, neuro and vascular surgeries.

Many drugs with ganglion blocking activity have been prepared and used clinically but only a few are still in use. It was hoped to develop agents which were, firstly, well absorbed orally and, secondly, specific for sympathetic ganglia in order to produce reliable blood pressure lowering effects and to reduce the spectrum of unwanted effects. Success was achieved with the former objective but not with the latter.

Ganglion blocking agents in current clinical use

Pentolinium (Pentolinium Tartrate BP)

pentolinium tartrate

Pentolinium is a bisquaternary compound and in most respects its actions closely resemble those of hexamethonium. It is slightly better absorbed orally than hexamethonium but produces a similar wide spectrum of side-effects and tolerance to its continued use often develops.

Clinical uses and dosage. Pentolinium tartrate finds occasional use to treat severe hypertension particularly when milder drugs have been tried and have failed. The usual starting dose is about

1 to 2·5 mg (subcutaneously) or 10 to 20 mg (orally). These doses may have to be increased up to 20 mg per day by the subcutaneous route and up to 900 mg per day orally to maintain adequate blood pressure control.

Pentolinium Injection (BP, BNF) contains 5 mg/ml of pentolinium tartrate and tablets (strength unspecified) receive official (BPC) recognition. It is commercially available as an injection containing 5 mg/ml and as tablets each containing 10 or 40 mg under the trade-name of ANSOLYSEN.

Mecamylamine

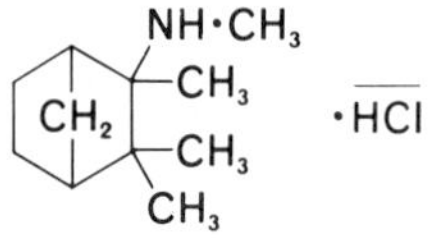

mecamylamine hydrochloride

This substance was introduced in 1956 (Stone, Torchiana, Navarro & Beyer) and was the first non-quaternary ganglion blocker to be used clinically. It is a secondary amine and is well absorbed by mouth and produces an antihypertensive effect lasting six to twelve hours. It produces the usual spectrum of side-effects as described for hexamethonium and additionally it penetrates into the brain and may cause unpleasant central side-effects, the most common of which is a tremor similar to that occurring in Parkinson's disease. However, more severe effects including mental confusion, seizures, mania and depression have been reported in occasional patients. Tolerance to the drug sometimes develops on prolonged use.

Clinical uses and dosage. Mecamylamine is sometimes used to control severe hypertension in patients refractory to other antihypertensive agents. It produces a reliable antihypertensive effect when given orally and starting doses of 2·5 mg twice daily are generally used and may be increased up to 60 mg daily if necessary. It is available as tablets containing either 2·5 or 10 mg under the trade-name of INVERSINE.

Pempidine

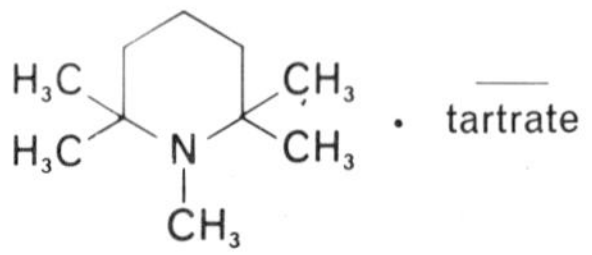

pempidine tartrate

Pempidine is a tertiary amine and represents the last genuine advance in this series of compounds. It was introduced in 1958 as a result of independent research by two separate pharmaceutical companies who arrived at its synthesis by different routes (Corn & Edge, 1958; Spinks, Young, Farrington & Dunlop, 1958). It is well absorbed by mouth but does not pass into the brain as readily as mecamylamine and is consequently less likely to cause central side-effects. Tolerance to its effects on prolonged administration is rare. However, it produces the spectrum of unwanted effects characteristic of this class of compound.

Clinical uses and dosage. For severe hypertension the usual starting dose is 2·5 mg orally every 6 hours increasing up to a maximum of 80 mg per day. It is commercially available as tablets each containing 1 or 5 mg of pempidine tartrate (PERO-LYSEN).

Trimetaphan

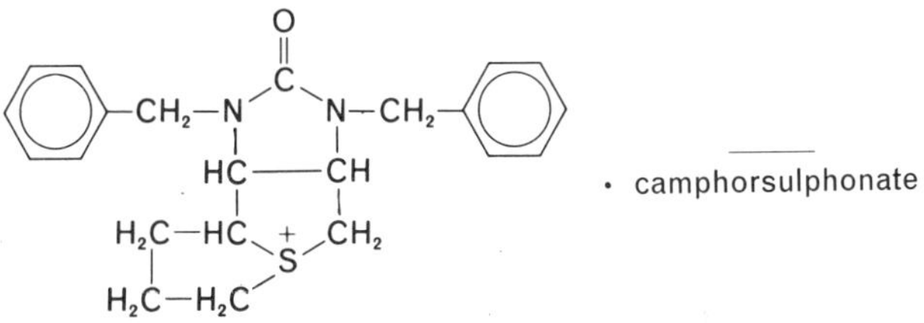

trimetaphan camphorsulphonate

Trimetaphan is a very short-acting ganglion blocker which is used to produce controlled hypotension during surgical procedures. The usual dose is 50 mg to 1 gram administered intravenously as a 0·1 per cent solution over a period of up to 2 hours. It is available commercially (ARFONAD) in ampoules each containing 250 mg of the dry solid packed with further ampoules containing 5 ml of Water for Injection.

Recent evidence regarding the transmission process in autonomic ganglia

As mentioned previously the concept of ganglionic transmission involving one neurotransmitter (acetylcholine) acting on one receptor type (nicotinic) is probably an over-simplification. Volle & Koelle (1975) have reviewed the evidence which suggests the existence of at least two other secondary pathways. In sympathetic ganglia acetylcholine produces a triphasic electrical response in the postsynaptic membrane. There is an initial excitatory postsynaptic potential (EPSP) which is followed in turn by an inhibitory postsynaptic potential (IPSP) and a late EPSP. The initial EPSP is blocked by hexamethonium but not by atropine and is thought to initiate the primary transmission process whilst the late EPSP is blocked by atropine but not by hexamethonium and is therefore thought to involve muscarinic receptors. The IPSP is blocked by α-adrenoreceptor blocking drugs and by atropine but not by hexamethonium. The usual interpretation of these facts is that the IPSP involves a neuronal pathway within the ganglion which utilises both α-adrenoreceptors and muscarinic receptors.

The physiological significance (if any) of these sites in sympathetic ganglia is not clear since atropine even in full doses does not produce detectable ganglion blockade, whereas hexamethonium is able to fully block the responses of a tissue, such as the cat's nictitating membrane, to preganglionic stimulation. Roskowski (1961) has described a compound (McN-A-343) which is a selective agonist for the muscarinic receptors in sympathetic ganglia and the effects of which are blocked by atropine. McN-A-343 produces responses, such as vasoconstriction, in whole animals which closely resemble the effects produced by stimulation of sympathetic nerves and which are abolished by drugs such as guanethidine (Chapter 10) which prevent the release of noradrenaline from sympathetic postganglionic nerves. These results suggest that the muscarinic receptors offer an alternative pathway for ganglionic transmission. Parasympathetic ganglia are much more difficult to examine experimentally since they are generally diffuse and inaccessible but indirect evidence using McN-A-343 suggests that they do not contain muscarinic receptors.

McN-A-343

Physiologically-occurring substances with actions at autonomic ganglia

In addition to muscarinic and nicotinic receptors for acetylcholine there is convincing evidence that autonomic ganglia contain receptors for catecholamines and for other substances. The naturally-occurring catecholamines noradrenaline, adrenaline and dopamine each cause hyperpolarisation of the post-synaptic membranes of ganglia with a consequent depression of transmission. These effects are abolished by α-adrenoreceptor blocking agents to reveal a facilitatory action, shared by the β-adrenoreceptor stimulant isoprenaline, and abolished by β-adrenoreceptor blocking agents. Thus both α and β adreno-receptors having opposing effects on the transmission process are present in autonomic ganglia. Histamine, 5-hydroxytrypt-amine and angiotensin II have also been shown to facilitate gang-lionic transmission by actions on their respective specific recep-tors. The physiological significance of these effects are not clear but they may be a reflection of an important role of autonomic ganglia in sorting physiological information of potential homeo-static value.

Classification of acetylcholine receptors

It is evident from the activity at autonomic ganglia of simple quaternary compounds such as TMA and TEA that the nicotinic receptor for acetylcholine has less stringent structural require-ments of the agonist than does the muscarinic receptor. TMA is a powerful nicotinic stimulant but has feeble activity at muscar-inic receptors. This is explained by postulating that the muscar-inic receptor has at least two major points of attachment (anionic and esteratic sites) whilst the ganglionic nicotinic receptor has only one (anionic) and hence only the quaternary group of acetylcholine is necessary for nicotinic stimulation. The action of bisquaternary compounds such as hexamethonium in blocking ganglionic transmission has been explained on the basis that the two positively charged nitrogen atoms may each combine with a nicotinic receptor simultaneously. A more likely explanation is that one cationic head combines with the anionic site of a nicotinic receptor whilst the other combines with an adjacent site, not part of the nicotinic receptor, which serves to 'anchor' the antagonist molecule in position.

There are marked differences in the effects of both agonists and antagonists at nicotinic receptors in autonomic ganglia when compared with their effects at nicotinic receptors at neuro-effector junctions in voluntary muscle. This may be explicable, in part, on differences in accessibility of the receptor sites to different agonists and antagonists. However, the bulk of the evidence suggests marked differences in the nature of the recep-tors at the two sites. There is similar evidence to suggest that neither nicotinic nor muscarinic receptors are homogenous populations. Thus the ganglion stimulant DMPP is much more effective in stimulating catecholamine release from the adrenal medullae than it is in stimulating sympathetic ganglia. Conversely, a compound ($N:N$-di-isopropyl-N^1-isopentyl-N^1-di-ethylamino-ethyl-urea) has been described which blocks cholinergic transmission in the adrenal medullae but is only feebly active in sympathetic ganglia. McN-A-343 which stimulates muscarinic receptors in sympathetic ganglia has little activity on muscarinic receptors in some other tissues.

In conclusion it must be emphasised that our present knowledge concerning drug-receptor interactions is very limited and current theories concerning the precise nature of these interactions and of the structure of receptors, do not satisfactorily explain all the available experimental data.

SUMMARY

The primary pathway for the transmission of nerve impulses in autonomic ganglia and in the cells of the adrenal medullae is via acetylcholine released from preganglionic nerve endings and acting upon nicotinic receptors in the postsynaptic membranes. The alkaloid nicotine first stimulates and then blocks autonomic ganglia. TMA and DMPP are potent ganglionic stimulants with less blocking activity than nicotine; they are used experimentally but have no clinical uses.

Autonomic ganglion blocking agents compete with acetylcholine for the nicotinic receptors in autonomic ganglia. These drugs are used clinically for their effects in blocking the ganglia of sympathetic vasoconstrictor nerves to blood vessels; they cause vasodilatation and a fall in blood pressure in patients suffering from hypertension. The ganglion blockers are equally effective at both sympathetic and parasympathetic ganglia and they therefore cause a wide spectrum of unwanted effects such as postural hypotension, atony of the bladder and intestine and impotence in the male. The earliest clinically useful drugs in this class were the bisquaternary compounds hexamethonium and pentolinium which suffer from the additional disadvantages of poor oral absorption and the development of tolerance on repeated dosage. Mecamylamine (secondary amine) and pempidine (tertiary amine) are more recently developed substances which are well absorbed orally but which have a tendency to produce unpleasant side-effects on the central nervous system in addition to the usual spectrum of peripheral effects.

The ganglion blocking agents have been largely replaced in the treatment of hypertension by more specific drugs but they are sometimes used to treat severe hypertension and also to produce controlled hypotension, in order to reduce bleeding, in some surgical procedures.

Recent research indicates that ganglionic transmission may be modified by a number of naturally-occurring substances such as noradrenaline, 5-hydroxytryptamine and angiotensin II all of which appear to have specific receptors within the ganglia. The physiological significance of these findings is, as yet, unclear.

REFERENCES

Acheson, G. H. & Moe, G. K. (1946) The action of tetraethyl ammonium ion on the mammalian circulation. *J. Pharmac. exp. Ther.*, **87**, 220–236.

Acheson, G. H. & Pereira, S. A. (1946) The blocking effect of tetraethylammonium ion on the superior cervical ganglion of the cat. *J. Pharmac. exp. Ther.*, **87**, 273–280.

Barlow, R. B. & Ing, H. R. (1948) Curare-like action of polymethylene bis-quaternary ammonium bases. *J. Pharmac. exp. Ther.*, **3**, 298–304.

Burn, J. H. & Dale, H. H. (1915) The action of certain quaternary ammonium bases. *J. Pharmac. exp. Ther.*, **6**, 417–438.

Corne, S. J. & Edge, N. D. (1958) Pharmacological properties of pempidine (1:2:2:6:6-pentamethyl piperidine) a new ganglion blocking compound. *Br. J. Pharmac.*, **13**, 339–349.

Langley, J. N. & Dickinson, W. L. (1889) On the local paralysis of peripheral ganglia, and on the connexion of different classes of nerve fibres with them. *Proc. R. Soc. B.*, **46**, 423–431.

Marshall, C. R. (1913) Studies on the pharmacological action of tetra-alkyl-ammonium compounds. *Trans. R. Soc. Edinb.*, **50**, Part I, 17–40, Part II, 379–396.

Morrison, B. M. & Paton, W. D. M. (1953) Effects of hexamethonium on normal individuals in relation to its concentration in the plasma. *Br. Med. J.*, **1**, 1299–1305.

Paton, W. D. M. & Zaimis, E. J. (1949) The pharmacological actions of polymethylene bistrimethylammonium salts. *Br. J. Pharmac.*, **4**, 381–400.

Roszkowski, A. P. (1961) An unusual type of sympathetic ganglionic stimulant. *J. Pharmac. exp. Ther.*, **132**, 156–170.

Spinks, A., Young, E. H. P., Farrington, J. A. & Dunlop, D. (1958) The pharmacological actions of pempidine and its ethyl homologue. *Br. J. Pharmac.*, **13**, 501–520.

Stone, C. A., Torchiana, M. L., Navarro, A. & Beyer, K. H. (1956) Ganglionic blocking properties of 3-methylamino-isocamphane hydrochloride (mecamylamine): A secondary amine. *J. Pharmac. exp. Ther.*, **117**, 169–183.

Volle, R. L. & Koelle, G. B. (1975) Ganglionic stimulating and blocking agents. In *The Pharmacological Basis of Therapeutics*, 5th edn., pp 565–574, (eds.) Goodman, L. S. & Gilman, A. New York: Macmillan Publishing Co.

GENERAL READING

Barlow, R. B. (1964) *Introduction to Chemical Pharmacology.* London: Menthuen & Co. Ltd.

Brimblecombe, R. W. (1974) *Drug Actions on Cholinergic Systems.* London: The Macmillan Press Ltd.

Gyermek, L. (1967) Ganglionic stimulant and depressant agents. In Drugs affecting the peripheral nervous system Vol. 1, pp 149–326. ed. Burger, A. London: Edward Arnold Ltd.

Ing, H. R. (1956) Structure-action relationships of hypotensive drugs. In *Hypotensive Drugs.* pp 7–22, ed. Harrington, M. Oxford: Pergamon Press.

Trendelenburg, U. (1967) Some aspects of the pharmacology of autonomic ganglion cells. *Ergebn. Physiol.*, **59,** 1–85.

Volle, R. L. (1966) Muscarinic and nicotinic stimulant actions at autonomic ganglia. In *International Encyclopedia of Pharmacology and Therapeutics.* Section 12, Vol. 1, ed. Karczmar, A. G. Oxford:Pergamon Press.

Volle, R. L. (1969) Ganglionic transmission. *A. Rev. Pharmac.*, **9,** 135–146.

8

Noradrenaline; its storage, synthesis, release and inactivation in the body

The evidence leading to the positive identification of noradrenaline as the neurotransmitter substance released from sympathetic (noradrenergic) nerves was reviewed in Chapter 3. The closely-related substance adrenaline is synthesised, stored and released from chromaffin cells present mainly in the adrenal medullae and from the much smaller number scattered throughout the body. The events occurring in noradrenergic nerves whereby noradrenaline is elaborated, stored and released have been the subject of intensive investigation, particularly in the last twenty or so years. The results of these investigations provide a wealth of fine detail which give the possibly erroneous impression that these events occurring in noradrenergic nerves are much more complex than analogous events occurring in cholinergic nerves. The reason for the greater research interest is noradrenergic rather than cholinergic neuronal mechanisms may be partly explained by the convenient model for catecholamine storage, synthesis and release mechanisms afforded by the large and accessible chromaffin cells of the adrenal medullae which were widely utilised in earlier studies. Another possible reason is the considerable therapeutic potential of drugs influencing sympathetic mechanisms in the treatment of important conditions such as hypertension.

ANATOMY OF NORADRENERGIC TERMINALS

Our knowledge of the detailed anatomy of noradrenergic nerves was scanty until the discovery by Falck, Hillarp, Thieme and Torp (1962) of a histochemical method for the direct visualisation of noradrenaline within noradrenergic neurones. The basis of the technique involves the condensation of catecholamines with formaldehyde vapour to form substances producing characteristic fluorescence when viewed by ultra-violet light. This elegant method has enabled a precise mapping of the noradrenergic innervation of many tissues to be made (see Fig. 8.1). Considerable advances have also been made by the use of the electron microscope particularly in the detailed examination of the junctions between noradrenergic neurones and smooth muscle effector cells (Fig. 8.2). The use of these techniques has caused many previous concepts regarding the structure and functioning of the fine terminations of noradren-

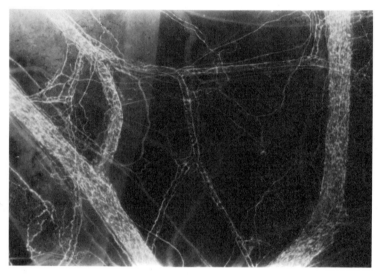

Fig. 8.1 Fluorescence photomicrograph of rat mesentery showing the strongly fluorescent plexus of varicose noradrenergic terminals surrounding the arterioles. (From D. R. Tomlinson, unpublished).

ergic nerves to be modified. For instance, much has been written about noradrenergic nerve endings when in fact viewed under the microscope free nerve endings are rarely seen. The structures involved in the innervation of effector cells by noradrenergic neurones consists of a dense network of very fine nerve fibres which derive from sympathetic nerve trunks by repeated branching and which have been called the *ground-plexus*. The synapses between nerve fibres and effector cells appear as swellings (*varicosities*) of the fine fibres giving them the characteristic bead-like appearance seen by fluorescent microscopy. The evidence from electron microscopy suggests that each noradrenergic fibre may make synaptic connections with many effector cells and conversely each effector cell may be innervated by many fibres arising from the same or different neurones.

Intraneuronal storage of noradrenaline

The experimental evidence from both biochemical and pharmacological investigations suggests that noradrenaline is stored within the neurone in two ways. Firstly, some is diffusely distributed throughout the cytoplasm of the cell in a loosely

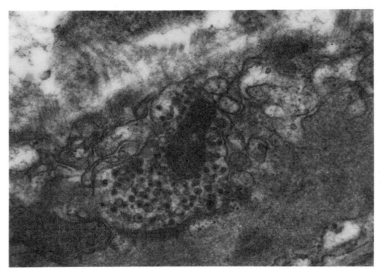

Fig. 8.2 Electron photomicrograph showing a noradrenergic nerve terminal varicosity in the smooth muscle of the rat vas deferens. The cytoplasm within the nerve terminal contains a mitochondrion and many vesicles some of which contain a densely stained core. Magnification approximately × 40 000. (From D. R. Tomlinson, unpublished).

bound form whilst the remainder is more tightly bound within granular vesicles many of which have a dense core and are concentrated in the varicosities of the ground-plexus. There is evidence to suggest that many of the larger noradrenaline-storage vesicles are formed in the cell bodies of noradrenergic neurones and pass along the axons by a process involving structures called microtubules to the varicosities. Within the storage vesicles noradrenaline is present in very high concentration and much evidence points to its being stored in the form of a molecular complex, probably with adenosine triphosphate

(ATP). Noradrenaline and ATP are present in the vesicles in constant stochiometric proportions of 4 molecules of noradrenaline to one molecule of ATP and disruption of the vesicles causes the release of both substances together with protein material which is also believed to be involved in the binding process.

Biosynthesis of noradrenaline and adrenaline

In 1939 Blaschko proposed a hypothetical series of reactions whereby noradrenaline and adrenaline might be formed in the body from the essential amino acid (−)-tyrosine. It was almost

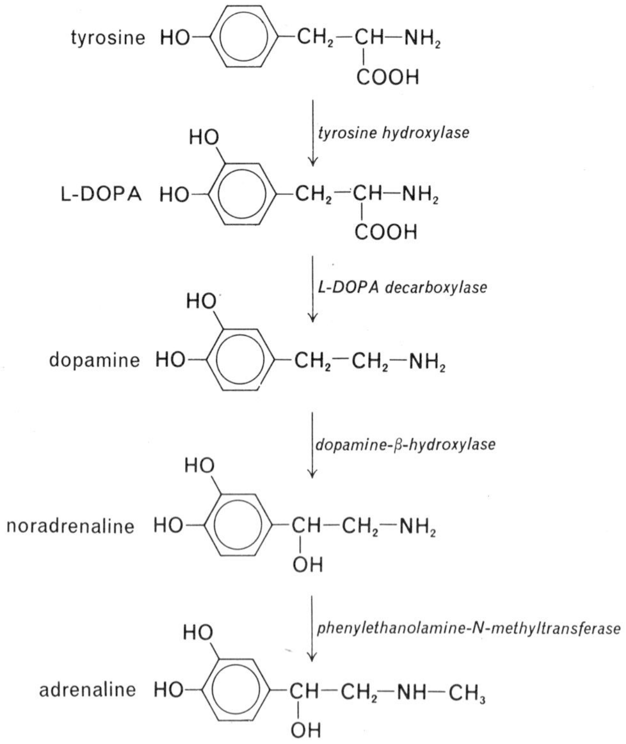

Fig. 8.3 Biosynthetic pathway for catecholamines. (−)-Tyrosine is taken up from the bloodstream by noradrenergic neurones and by the chromaffin cells of the adrenal medullae. In noradrenergic nerves the conversion of tyrosine to L-DOPA and of L-DOPA to dopamine occurs in the cytoplasm of the neurone; dopamine is then taken into the noradrenaline storage vesicles where conversion to noradrenaline takes place. The conversion of noradrenaline to adrenaline does not occur in noradrenergic nerves but takes place in those chromaffin cells of the adrenal medullae which store adrenaline.

20 years before this brilliantly conceived pathway was verified in experiments initially using chromaffin cells of the adrenal medullae and subsequently in others using homogenates of sympathetic nerves and ganglia. The pathway for the synthesis of (−)-noradrenaline and (−)-adrenaline from (−)-tyrosine is shown in Fig. 8.3. (−)-Tyrosine is present in ample amounts in any balanced diet and may additionally be synthesised in the body from the related amino acid (−)-phenylalanine. Tyrosine is taken up by noradrenergic nerves and by chromaffin tissue and the same synthetic pathway is followed at each site terminating with (−)-noradrenaline in noradrenergic nerves and with (−)-adrenaline in those chromaffin cells which produce and store adrenaline. In noradrenergic nerves the enzymes tyrosine hydroxylase and L-DOPA decarboxylase are present in the cytoplasm and synthesis as far as dopamine occurs outside of the noradrenaline storage vesicles. Dopamine is actively taken up by the vesicles and its conversion to noradrenaline occurs within the vesicles in the presence of dopamine β-hydroxylase. Since noradrenaline is not synthesised within the cytoplasm of the neurones it follows that the cytoplasmic pool of noradrenaline must arise either from transfer or leakage from the granules or more probably as a result of active uptake of preformed noradrenaline from extra-neuronal sites. The rate-limiting step for noradrenaline synthesis is probably the tyrosine to L-DOPA stage which is catalysed by tyrosine hydroxylase and inhibited by noradrenaline providing what is known as *end-product inhibition* and which thus controls the rate of noradrenaline production.

Noradrenergic nerves are not readily depleted of their noradrenaline stores by prolonged electrical stimulation even when high stimulus frequencies are used. This suggests that stimulation is probably able to increase synthesis and/or re-uptake (see later) of noradrenaline. The rapid loss of noradrenaline occurring during prolonged stimulation would also tend to reduce the end-product inhibition of tyrosine hydroxylase by noradrenaline.

Production of Adrenaline from noradrenaline

Noradrenergic nerves do not contain the enzyme phenyl-ethanolamine-N-methyltransferase (PNMT) necessary for the production of adrenaline from noradrenaline. This enzyme is present in the adrenaline-producing cells of the adrenal medullae but not in those chromaffin cells producing noradrenaline. Recent evidence suggests that the enzyme may be present in the mammalian brain and therefore opens the possibility of true adrenergic (i.e. adrenaline-releasing) neurones occurring in mammals.

Inhibitors of catecholamine synthesis

The enzymes involved in all stages of the biosynthesis of catecholamines have been characterised and specific inhibitors of each have been described. However, thus far few clinical uses have been found for these substances. Inhibitors of L-DOPA decarboxylase such as benserazide (Ro4-4602) are used to prevent the peripheral side-effects due to dopamine formation in patients given L-DOPA for the treatment of Parkinsonism. Parkinson's disease is characterised by reduced amounts of dopamine in the corpus striatum of the brain and often striking benefit can be gained by recharging these stores by the administration of L-DOPA the precursor of dopamine. Benserazide does not penetrate into the brain appreciably and so does not interfere with the central conversion of L-DOPA to dopamine.

α-methylDOPA (ALDOMET) is a competitive inhibitor of L-DOPA decarboxylase and is an important drug in the treatment of hypertension (see Chapter 13). However, the clinical effect of this substance is not directly related to inhibition of this enzyme. Dopamine-β-hydroxylase is inhibited by disulfiram (ANTABUSE), a substance used clinically to treat alcoholism. However, the useful effect in alcoholism is not due to inhibition of dopamine-β-hydroxylase but to preventing the complete oxidation of ethanol leading to unpleasant symptoms due to the build-up of acetaldehyde in the body.

Release of noradrenaline on neuronal stimulation

Releatively little is known about the events which promote the release of noradrenaline from the terminal varicosities of noradrenergic nerves and even less about the events which couple secretion of transmitter with responses in effector cells. The bulk of the available evidence suggests that stimulus-secretion coupling in noradrenergic nerves is basically similar to that occurring in chromaffin cells and in cholinergic neurones. As in cholinergic nerves, at rest there is a small, apparently random, release of transmitter from the varicosities which induces characteristic small electrical changes in the post-synaptic cells. On passage of an action potential down the axon many vesicles release their content of noradrenaline into the gap (*synaptic cleft*) between the terminal varicosity and the effector cell. The process whereby the noradrenaline-containing storage vesicles migrate to the plasma membrane, become structurally-attached to it and liberate their contents is called *exocytosis* and is illustrated diagramatically in Fig. 8.4. Exocytosis is dependent on the influx of calcium ions into the terminal region of the noradrenergic nerve. The precise role of calcium in the noradrenaline-release process is not known but it has been suggested that intracellular calcium ions are necessary for the attachment of the storage vesicles to the inner surface of the neuronal plasma membrane. After discharge of their contents it is thought that most of the outer membranes of the storage vesicles are retained within the neurone and may possibly be re-used for manufacture of small storage vesicles which are then refilled with noradrenaline from the cytoplasmic pool.

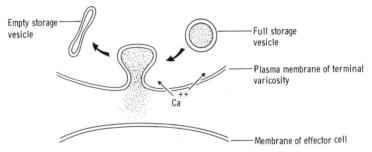

Fig. 8.4 Diagrammatic representation of the release of noradrenaline from storage vesicles in noradrenergic nerves by exocytosis. On excitation of the cell and during the inflow of calcium ions the full storage vesicles become attached to the plasma membrane of the terminal varicosities and discharge their contents into the synaptic clefts. The empty storage vesicles are retained by the neurone and may possibly be refilled with noradrenaline.

Influence of stimulus frequency on noradrenaline release

When their sympathetic nerves are electrically stimulated most tissues respond to stimulus frequencies as low as one impulse per second (*one Herz*) and some, such as the nictitating membrane of the cat, will respond when the nerves are stimulated with a single impulse. Most sympathetically-innervated tissues show a marked change in responsiveness over the stimulus range of 1–5 Herz and maximal responses are usually obtained at frequencies between 20–40 Herz (see Fig. 8.5). The work of Folkow (1952) suggests that the rate of firing in noradrenergic nerves in man rarely exceeds 10 Herz and is usually in the range of only 1–2 Herz. With stimulus frequencies in excess of 10–20 Herz the output of noradrenaline per stimulus declines.

Presynaptic receptors modulating neuronal release of noradrenaline

Recent work, particularly by S. Z. Langer and his colleagues (Langer, 1977) suggests that in addition to adrenoreceptors in effector cells activated by noradrenaline released from postganglionic sympathetic nerves there also exists presynaptic adrenoreceptors on the varicosities themselves which may modulate transmitter release. During moderate activity of

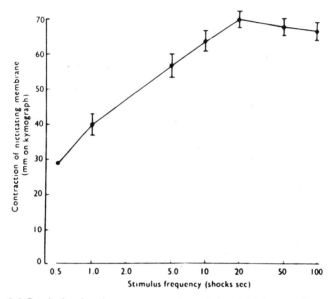

Fig. 8.5 Graph showing the mean contractions of the nictitating membranes in a group of 4 cats in response to postganglionic stimulation of the cervical sympathetic nerve with 200 pulses at the frequencies indicated. (From Day & Rand, 1964).

postganglionic noradrenergic nerves some of the noradrenaline released diffuses back from postsynaptic sites and activates presynaptic α-adrenoreceptors which in turn diminish the output per stimulus of transmitter thus forming a negative feed-back system. Similarly, in situations where the neuronal output of noradrenaline is low it is thought that some of it combines with presynaptic β-adrenoreceptors which promote an increased output per stimulus of noradrenaline.

There is other evidence to suggest that presynaptic receptors modulating noradrenaline release also exist for a number of other substances including dopamine, angiotensin II and prostaglandins. There may well be similar presynaptic receptors in postganglionic parasympathetic nerves whose role is to modulate acetylcholine release. The presence of these presynaptic receptors is reminiscent of the receptors present in autonomic ganglia (see Chapter 7) which likewise may have a physiological role to play in the fine control of the peripheral autonomic nervous system.

Biological inactivation of noradrenaline

The inactivation of noradrenaline released from noradrenergic nerves and from the adrenal medullae is a complex process involving both enzymatic destruction and physical removal of unchanged noradrenaline molecules from biologically-active extraneuronal sites to inactive sites within the neurone. Much of the early work concerning the biological inactivation of catecholamines was influenced by the search for an enzymatic counterpart in the noradrenergic system to acetylcholinesterase in the cholinergic system. However, as Gillespie (1973) has pointed out, acetylcholine serves solely as a neurotransmitter substance and hence its rapid destruction is desirable to prevent widespread effects whereas noradrenaline when released from the adrenal medullae functions as a hormone and its over-rapid destruction would in these circumstances render it ineffective.

Monoamine Oxidase

An enzyme which oxidatively deaminated tyramine was discovered in mammalian liver by Hare (1928) and was later shown to also destroy adrenaline (Blaschko, Richter and Schlossman, 1937). The enzyme was called 'amine oxidase' by Richter (1937) and this name was later modified to monoamine oxidase to distinguish it from another group of enzymes present in the body which similarly attack diamines. Monoamine oxidase oxidizes the catecholamines dopamine, noradrenaline and adrenaline in the body to inactive substances (Fig. 8.6); it also attacks the biogenic amine 5-hydroxytryptamine. In the absence of a specific inhibitor for monoamine oxidase it was at first thought to serve a similar function in destroying catecholamines released from noradrenergic nerves and the adrenal medullae to that served by acetylcholinesterase in terminating the effects of acetylcholine released from cholinergic nerves. This view had to be discarded when, in the early 1950's, highly specific inhibitors of monoamine oxidase such as iproniazid were developed which, even in full enzyme-inhibiting doses, produced only marginal increases in the effects of noradrenergic nerve stimulation and of

injected noradrenaline in animal experiments. These observations clearly indicated the existence of an alternative route or
routes for the degradation of catecholamines. Despite this
observation there is much experimental evidence to suggest that
monoamine oxidase has a very important physiological role and
its inhibition in the brain by non-competitive inhibitors such as
iproniazid has been shown to be of value in the treatment of
severe mental depression. The enzyme is widely distributed in

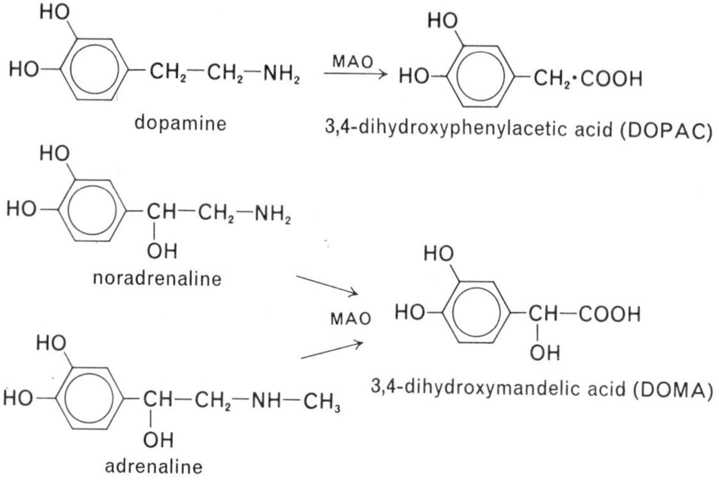

Fig. 8.6 Metabolites of dopamine, noradrenaline and adrenaline produced by
the action of monoamine oxidase (MAO).

the body, liver and kidney being rich sources, but the important
location in relation to its role in metabolising noradrenaline is
that found in the mitochondria within noradrenergic neurones.
Intraneuronal monoamine oxidase appears to be concerned with
the regulation of the size of the loosely-bound cytoplasmic
noradrenaline pool. Once noradrenaline is incorporated into the
storage vesicles it is protected from the action of the enzyme. In
many tissues following inhibition of monoamine oxidase the
concentration of intraneuronal noradrenaline is markedly
increased but despite this responses of effector tissues to stimulation of their noradrenergic nerves are little affected and may
even be slightly decreased. This suggests that the amount of
noradrenaline released by nerve stimuli is not directly related to
the level of endogenous noradrenaline and this view is supported
by the finding that neuronal noradrenaline stores have to be
depleted by 90 per cent or more before any marked reduction of

nerve-mediated responses in effector tissues occurs. Only a small proportion of the noradrenaline released on stimulation of noradrenergic nerves is metabolised by monoamine oxidase but a higher proportion of that released from the adrenal medullae and after therapeutic administration is metabolised in this way. The enzyme is of prime importance in degrading monoamines such as phenylethylamine and tyramine which may be taken in the diet or formed in the body as a result of the decarboxylation of the corresponding amino-acids. After inhibition of mono-amine oxidase these substances may reach levels in the body where they become biologically active as sympathomimetic substances and may induce dangerous increases in arterial blood pressure in patients treated with monoamine oxidase inhibitors to alleviate depression. This potentially lethal effect will be described more fully in the next chapter.

It is not clear whether monoamine oxidase inhibitors relieve depressive illness by increasing intraneuronal levels of noradren-aline within the brain or whether their effects in increasing central levels of 5-hydroxytryptamine and/or dopamine are of greater importance. Recent evidence suggests that monoamine oxidase exists in multiple forms having differing substrate specificities and distributions. This finding holds out hope that selective inhibitors of the various forms will be found leading to a greater understanding of the physiological role of these enzymes and perhaps to further therapeutic uses for their inhibitors.

Catechol-O-methyltransferase

Following the observed lack of effect on responses to noradren-ergic nerve stimulation and to noradrenaline produced by inhibition of monoamine oxidase a search was made for alter-native enzymatic pathways for the degradation of noradrenaline and other naturally-occurring catecholamines. This search culminated in the discovery by Axelrod (1957) of an enzyme which catalysed the transfer of a methyl group from S-adenosyl methionine to the meta hydroxy (3-position) group of catechol-amines. The enzyme system which requires the presence of magnesium ions has been called catechol-O-methyltransferase (COMT) and like monoamine oxidase it is widely distributed in the body and is present in considerable quantities in the kidneys and liver. However, unlike monoamine oxidase, it is not present inside noradrenergic neurones. The O-methylated metabolite of noradrenaline is called *normetanephrine*, that of adrenaline *metanephrine,* and that of dopamine *methoxytyramine* (Fig. 8.7). The enzymes catechol-O-methyltransferase and monoamine oxidase may act sequentially on catecholamines thus producing the further metabolites shown in Fig. 8.8. The available evidence suggests that O-methylation is not an important route for the metabolism of neuronally released noradrenaline whereas it is of major importance for terminating the effects of circulating catecholamines arising either from the

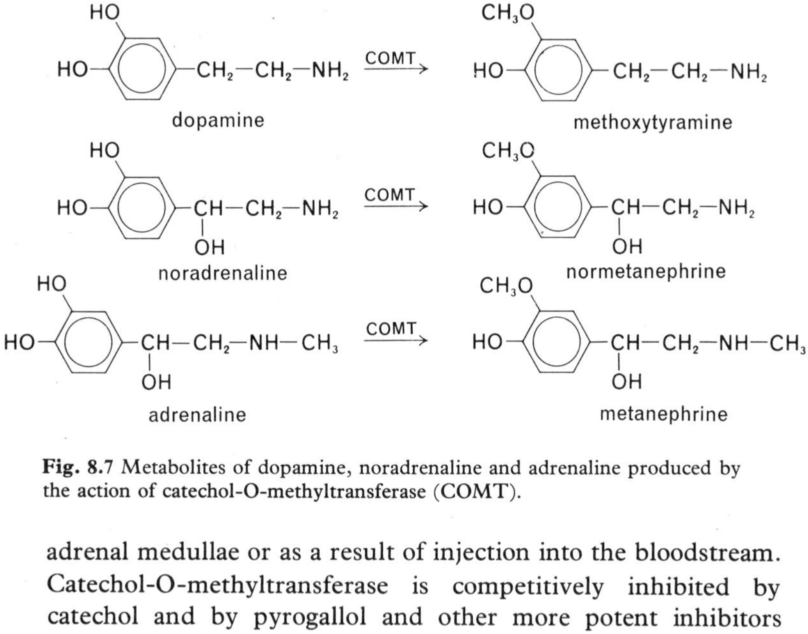

Fig. 8.7 Metabolites of dopamine, noradrenaline and adrenaline produced by the action of catechol-O-methyltransferase (COMT).

adrenal medullae or as a result of injection into the bloodstream. Catechol-O-methyltransferase is competitively inhibited by catechol and by pyrogallol and other more potent inhibitors have been described. Thus far no clinical use has been described for these substances and the precise role of catechol-O-methyltransferase in the body has probably yet to be determined.

Crout (1961) showed that in anaesthetised cats the simultaneous inhibition of monoamine oxidase and catechol-O-methyltransferase did not greatly increase either the height or the duration of pressor responses to intravenous catecholamines thus suggesting the existence of yet another major mechanism for terminating the biological effects of these substances.

The neuronal uptake process for noradrenaline (Uptake₁)

In 1910 Frohlich and Loewi reported that the pressor responses evoked by intravenously administered adrenaline were considerably augmented after the administration of cocaine. Some years later the plausible explanation was offered that this effect was due to the action of cocaine in competitively inhibiting monoamine oxidase. However, this view became untenable when in the 1950's it was discovered that much more potent inhibitors of this enzyme, such as iproniazid, did not produce a similar effect. Macmillan (1959) observed that the vasoconstrictor effects of sympathetic stimulation and of noradrenaline were

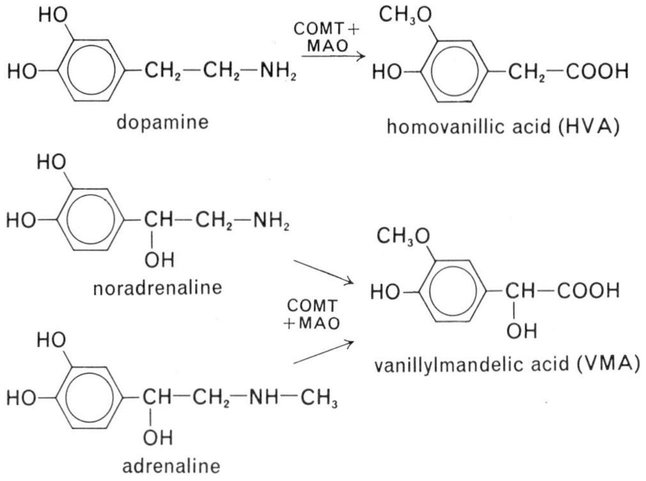

Fig. 8.8 Metabolites of dopamine, noradrenaline and adrenaline produced by combined action of catechol-O-methyltransferase (COMT) and monoamine oxidase (MAO).

greatly increased after an injection of cocaine (see Fig. 8.9). He suggested that cocaine was preventing the uptake of noradrenaline into the tissues and thus increasing its effective concentration at the receptors leading to increased responses. This suggestion was soon confirmed by the direct experiments of Whitby, Axelrod and Weil-Malherbe (1961) using radioactively labelled noradrenaline. These workers showed that many tissues in the cat took up noradrenaline from the bloodstream and the effect was greatest in those tissues such as the heart which have a rich sympathetic innervation. In similar experiments it was later shown that the uptake process was inhibited by cocaine and by degeneration of the noradrenergic nerves following either surgical or chemical sympathectomy. The loss of the neuronal uptake process for noradrenaline by sympathectomy produced a convincing explanation for the well-known supersensitivity of denervated tissues to noradrenaline. The neuronal uptake process for noradrenaline has been called Uptake$_1$ by Iversen to distinguish it from the non-neuronal noradrenaline uptake system which has also been described and which has been called Uptake$_2$ (Iversen, 1965).

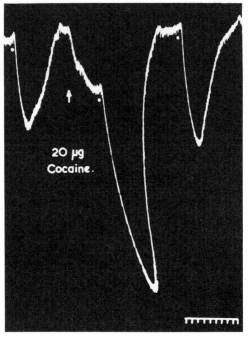

Fig. 8.9 Effect of cocaine on the vasoconstrictor action of noradrenaline. Venous outflow from isolated rabbit ear perfused with Locke solution. At the white dots 2 nanogram (ng) doses of noradrenaline were injected into the arterial cannula and caused vasoconstrictor responses which were greatly increased after the injection of cocaine (20 micrograms (μg) at the arrow). (Taken from Macmillan, 1959).

Properties of Uptake$_1$

The properties of Uptake$_1$ have been intensively studied in a variety of tissues and it appears that noradrenergic neurones both in the central nervous system and peripherally have an apparently identical process for concentrating noradrenaline and some related substances from the extra-cellular fluid. The uptake process is energy-dependent, is able to operate against a large concentration gradient, is saturable and has a high affinity for noradrenaline. In most tissues that have been studied

Uptake$_1$ is stereoselective having an affinity for the naturally-occurring ($-$)-noradrenaline some five times greater than for the ($+$)-isomer. In common with other membrane transport systems for organic compounds Uptake$_1$ is temperature sensitive and may be inhibited by some 50 per cent for each 10 °C drop in temperature below 37 °C. Uptake$_1$ is also dependent on the presence of both sodium ions and low concentrations (approximately 5 mM) of potassium ions. Concentrations of potassium ions above about 50 mM inhibit Uptake$_1$

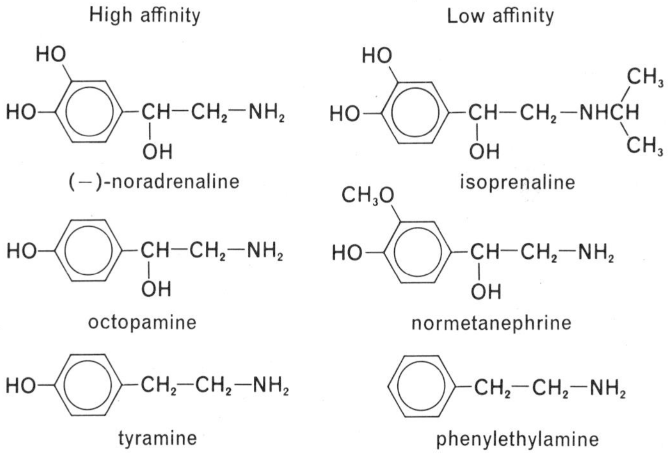

Fig. 8.10 Structural requirements for sympathomimetics to be transported by Uptake$_1$.
Substitution on the nitrogen atom reduces affinity; ($-$)-noradrenaline is transported whilst isoprenaline is not. Presence of methoxy groups on the aromatic ring reduces affinity such that ($-$)-noradrenaline and octopamine are substrates for Uptake$_1$ but normetanephrine is not. At least one hydroxyl group must be present on the benzene ring for transport by Uptake$_1$ thus tyramine is more readily transported than phenylethylamine.

In mammalian species the affinity of Uptake$_1$ for noradrenaline is approximately twice that for adrenaline. A number of other derivatives of phenylethylamine may be transported by Uptake$_1$ subject to certain structural requirements (see Fig. 8.10). Firstly, for rapid transport by Uptake$_1$ there must be no bulky substituent on the nitrogen atom; noradrenaline is readily transported whereas N-isopropylnoradrenaline (isoprenaline) is not. Secondly, the presence of a methoxy group on the aromatic ring reduces transport by Uptake$_1$; octopamine is readily transported but the 3-methoxy metabolite of noradrenaline (normetanephrine) is not. Finally, only those substances with at least one phenolic hydroxyl group on the aromatic ring are readily transported; tyramine is taken up by Uptake$_1$ much more readily than is phenylethylamine.

Physiological role of Uptake$_1$

Most of the evidence available points conclusively to Uptake$_1$ as being the most important mechanism whereby neuronally released noradrenaline is biologically inactivated. Although estimates vary it is likely that Uptake$_1$ accounts for the inactivation of between 75 and 90 per cent of the noradrenaline released by noradrenergic nerves.

Inhibitors of Uptake$_1$

A wide range of substances inhibit Uptake$_1$ and many of these substances produce an increase in the effects of exogenously administered noradrenaline and of the effects of noradrenergic nerve stimulation. Cocaine and the tricyclic antidepressant drugs, such as desmethylimipramine, are potent inhibitors of Uptake$_1$ at both central and peripheral sites. Peripherally these substances increase responses to injected noradrenaline and to sympathetic stimulation and their mood-elevating effects in the brain are believed to be due to the increased levels of noradrenaline at receptor sites which inhibition of Uptake$_1$ produces. Many compounds structurally related to phenylethylamine, but not conforming to the structural requirements for rapid transport by Uptake$_1$, are nevertheless attached to the Uptake$_1$ mechanism and may inhibit it. Examples of such substances are amphetamine, ephedrine and phenylethylamine. These substances tend to increase responses to sympathetic stimulation and also to substances normally more readily transported by Uptake$_1$. Noradrenergic neurone blocking drugs such as guanethidine and bethanidine (see Chapter 10) are potent inhibitors of Uptake$_1$. These substances prevent neuronal release of noradrenaline by a mechanism which is not completely understood but which appears to involve combination with the Uptake$_1$ mechanism and probably also transport by Uptake$_1$ to an intraneuronal site. Drugs such as amphetamine with a strong affinity for Uptake$_1$ but which are only slowly transported by it antagonise the action of the noradrenergic neurone blockers in preventing noradrenaline release.

Other neuronal catecholamine uptake processes
In the frog and toad where adrenaline is the sympathetic neurotransmitter the neuronal catecholamine uptake mechanism has been modified such that adrenaline is more readily taken up than noradrenaline. Similarly, in those areas of the mammalian brain where dopamine is a neurotransmitter the neuronal uptake process transports dopamine more readily than noradrenaline.

Uptake of catecholamines by storage vesicles
The processes whereby noradrenaline or related substance is transported from the cytoplasm of the neurone to the storage vesicle appears to be very similar to the process whereby substances are taken up by the storage granules of the chromaffin cells of the adrenal medullae. These uptake processes differ in several respects from $Uptake_1$. The vesicle uptake process has different structural requirements from $Uptake_1$, the presence of either a catechol or an alcoholic hydroxyl group being necessary. Thus dopamine and octopamine are taken up into storage vesicles whilst tyramine is not. Similarly, inhibitors of $Uptake_1$ have little effect on the uptake of substances into vesicles whereas the alkaloid reserpine which has little effect on $Uptake_1$ is a potent inhibitor of the vesicle uptake process.

Extraneuronal uptake of catecholamines ($Uptake_2$)

In addition to the specific neuronal uptake mechanisms for noradrenaline and related substances an extraneuronal uptake mechanism has been described by Iversen (1965) and named $Uptake_2$. This transport system occurs in various peripheral tissues including cardiac muscle and the smooth muscle of the blood vessels and of the intestine. $Uptake_2$ appears to operate only when high concentrations of catecholamines are circulating in the bloodstream and it also differs from $Uptake_1$ in several other important respects. Thus $Uptake_2$ has a higher maximum capacity for catecholamines but has a relatively lower affinity for noradrenaline and adrenaline and, unlike $Uptake_1$, is able to transport considerable quantities of isoprenaline. $Uptake_2$ does not exhibit any stereo preference and is not inhibited by $Uptake_1$ inhibitors. Following transport by $Uptake_2$ catecholamines are not stored but are rapidly metabolized intracellularly by both catechol-O-methyltransferase and monoamine oxidase.

The physiological significance, if any, of $Uptake_2$ is not clear but it has been suggested that it may play a role in the inactivation of catecholamines released from the adrenal medullae.

ADRENORECEPTORS, GENERAL CLASSIFICATION INTO α AND β TYPES

Terminology

Various terms have been used to describe the receptors on effector tissues with which catecholamines combine to initiate responses. The term 'adrenergic' was introduced by Dale to describe sympathetic nerves which released adrenaline or a related substance as a neurotransmitter. This choice of term, as previously mentioned, was a little unfortunate since it is now known that the large majority of mammalian postganglionic sympathetic nerves in fact release noradrenaline and not adrenaline; in the present monograph 'noradrenergic' has been used to describe these nerves. The confusion in the terminology has been compounded in recent years by many authors who have applied the term 'adrenergic' to receptors within the sympathetic system and also to agonists and antagonists of these receptors. Recently there has been some move towards rationalisation of the terminology and the terms adrenoreceptor and adrenoceptor have been coined to describe receptors for sympathomimetic substances. In the present monograph the term adrenoreceptor will be used throughout to describe receptors activated by sympathomimetic substances and the terms adrenoreceptor stimulant for agonist drugs and adrenoreceptor blocking agent for antagonists.

Classification of adrenoreceptors

Since the classic experiments of Oliver and Schäffer (1895) it has been known that the effects produced in the body by adrenaline in many ways resemble the effects produced by activating sympathetic nerves. For instance, adrenaline stimulates the rate and force of the heart beat and inhibits motility of the gastrointestinal tract. However, the reason why adrenaline stimulates smooth muscle in one tissue and inhibits it in another remained a mystery for many years. In 1906, Dale reported that in the anaesthetised cat certain preparations of extracts of the fungus ergot changed the effects produced by intravenously administered adrenaline from a rise in arterial blood pressure to a fall. Dale did not attempt an interpretation of this fascinating observation in terms of receptors although the conceptual groundwork for a receptor theory had been laid the previous year by Langley (1905). Langley, in attempting to explain the differing effects of adrenaline in various tissues, suggested that different 'receptive substances' (i.e. receptors) were present in tissues in which adrenaline produced an excitatory effect from those in which its effects were inhibitory. The observation was re-examined many years later by Cannon and Rosenblueth (1933) who were particularly concerned with the nature of the transmitter substance released by sympathetic nerves in tissues activated by sympathetic impulses compared with those which were inhibited. They hypothesised that a single transmitter substance (thought at the time to be probably adrenaline) was released by all sympathetic nerves and that this then combined with another substance in or near the effector cell to produce either an excitatory or an inhibitory transmitter. These modified transmitters Cannon and Rosenblueth called Sympathin E (excitor effects) and Sympathin I (inhibitory effects). The major flaw in the hypothesis was that transmitter taken from a tissue showing excitatory effects (Sympathin E) did not excite tissues in which sympathetic impulses were normally inhibitory but in fact was without effect or even inhibited them. This observation was much more in accord with Langley's earlier suggestion of differing receptors rather than differing transmitter substances. The modern view is based upon the classification of adrenoreceptors suggested by Ahlquist (1948). This worker studied the effects produced by adrenaline, noradrenaline and isoprenaline (also the α-methyl derivatives of adrenaline and noradrenaline) on a range of tissues taken from four mammalian species. It was found that the various responses fell into either of two major classes. In the first class adrenaline was the most powerful agonist and isoprenaline the least and in the second class isoprenaline was the most potent and noradrenaline the least. Ahlquist suggested that the two sets of responses reflected actions mediated by different sets of adrenoreceptors which he designated alpha (α) for the first type and beta (β) for the second. In general, α-adrenoreceptors mediate excitatory effects such as vasoconstriction, contraction of the smooth muscle of the uterus and vas deferens whilst β-adrenoreceptors subserve inhibitory effects such as vasodilatation and relaxation of the smooth muscle of the respiratory tract and detrusor muscle of the bladder. There are two major exceptions to this simple classification of α-excitatory and β-inhibitory adrenoreceptors; the α-adrenoreceptors in the gastrointestinal tract subserve inhibition of tone and motility of the smooth muscle (as do the β-adrenoreceptors which are also present in this tissue) and in cardiac muscle the adrenoreceptors which mediate increases in cardiac force and rate are of the β-type.

It follows from Ahlquist's work that adrenoreceptor agonists may stimulate one or other type of adrenoreceptor preferentially or, like adrenaline, stimulate both types. Thus, in general, noradrenaline has mainly α-adrenoreceptor stimulant activity whilst isoprenaline is practically specific for β-adrenoreceptors. The only structural requirement to add β-adrenoreceptor agonist potency to the noradrenaline molecule is substitution of alkyl groups on the nitrogen atom. Thus, adrenaline is N-methylnoradrenaline and isoprenaline N-isopropylnoradrenaline. There are a number of apparent paradoxes in the Ahlquist classification such as the reason for mammalian cardiac sympathetic nerves releasing noradrenaline as the transmitter substance when it appears not to be the most suitable agonist for β-adrenoreceptors. However, despite criticism of this sort, the classification has been of great value as a framework into which many experimental observations may be fitted. The theory has needed modification in detail with the passage of time and recently sub-groupings of both α and β-adrenoreceptors have been proposed and have been backed by experimental evidence. These modifications of the Ahlquist classification will be discussed in the following chapters in discussing the actions of α and β-adrenoreceptor agonists and antagonists.

SUMMARY

Postganglionic noradrenergic nerve fibres branch repeatedly to give rise to a ground plexus having a characteristic beaded appearance when viewed under the microscope. The beaded portions of the fibres are called terminal varicosities and are believed to be the site of synthesis, storage and release of the transmitter substance noradrenaline. Noradrenaline is synthesised intraneuronally from the amino-acid $(-)$ tyrosine which is taken up from the bloodstream and converted enzymatically to noradrenaline via the synthetic pathway $(-)$ tyrosine $\rightarrow$ $(-)$ DOPA $\rightarrow$ dopamine $\rightarrow$ $(-)$ noradrenaline. In some chromaffin cells of the adrenal medullae the synthetic pathway proceeds to adrenaline. Noradrenaline is stored intraneuronally in specialised storage vesicles which, on stimulation of the nerve, release their contents into the synaptic cleft by a process known as exocytosis involving the influx of calcium ions into the terminal varicosities and combination of the storage vesicles with the plasma membrane of the nerve fibre.

Noradrenaline released from sympathetic nerves is partly inactivated by metabolism by the enzyme systems monoamine oxidase (oxidative deamination) and catechol-O-methyltransferase (methylation of the hydroxyl group in the 3-position on the benzene ring). However, it is likely that more than 75 per cent of neuronally-released noradrenaline is inactivated by re-uptake into the neurone for subsequent re-use as transmitter. Monoamine oxidase and catechol-O-methyltransferase are widely distributed in the body but only monoamine oxidase is present within the mitochondria of noradrenergic neurones. It appears that monoamine oxidase has an important role in regulating the amount of noradrenaline stored intraneuronally whilst the most important function of catechol-O-methyl-transferase is inactivation by methylation of circulating catecholamines. The neuronal uptake mechanism for catecholamines (Uptake$_1$) is an energy-dependent membrane transport system which is able to transport noradrenaline and some structurally related substances into the neurone. Uptake$_1$ is both stereo and structure selective having a higher affinity for $(-)$ than $(+)$ noradrenaline and a very low affinity for isoprenaline. Uptake$_1$ is inhibited by a number of substances including cocaine, tricyclic compounds such as imipramine and some sympathomimetic substances such as dexamphetamine.

Noradrenaline released from sympathetic nerves produces its characteristic effects in effector tissues by combining with adrenoreceptors in the effector cells. Adrenoreceptors have been classified into two main types called α and β. α-adrenoreceptors, in general, subserve the excitatory effects of noradrenaline such as vasoconstriction and contraction of the smooth muscle of the spleen and vas deferentia. β-adrenoreceptors mainly subserve inhibitory responses such as relaxation of bronchial and intestinal smooth muscle. However, there are exceptions to this broad classification of α-excitor and β-inhibitory effects; α-adreno-receptors present in the gastrointestinal tract have an inhibitory function whilst the β-adrenoreceptors of the heart subserve excitatory effects.

REFERENCES

Ahlquist, R. P. (1948) A study of adrenotropic receptors. *Am. J. Physiol.*, **153,** 586–600.

Axelrod, J. (1957) 0–Methylation of epinephrine and other catechols in vitro and in vivo. *Science*, **126,** 400–401.

Blaschko, H. (1939) The specific action of L-DOPA decarboxylase. *J. Physiol.*, **96**, 50–51P.

Blaschko, H., Richter, D. & Schlossman, H. (1937) The oxidation of adrenaline and other amines. *Biochem. J.*, **31**, 2187–2196.

Cannon, W. B. & Rosenblueth, A. (1933) Sympathin E and sympathin I. *Am. J. Physiol.*, **104**, 557–574.

Crout, J. R. (1961) Effect of inhibiting both catechol-0-methyltransferase and monoamine oxidase on cardiovascular responses to norepinephrine. *Proc. Soc. exp. Biol. Med.*, **108**, 482–484.

Dale, H. H. (1906) On some physiological actions of ergot. *J. Physiol.*, **34**, 163–206.

Day, M. D. & Rand, M. J. (1964) Some observations on the pharmacology of α-methyldopa. *Br. J. Pharmac.*, **22**, 72–86.

Falk, B., Hillarp, N. A., Thieme, G. & Torp, A. (1962) Fluorescence of catecholamines and related compounds condensed with formaldehyde. *J. Histochem. Cytochem.*, **10**, 348–354.

Folkow, B. (1952) Impulse frequency in sympathetic vasomotor fibres correlated to the release and elimination of the transmitter. *Acta physiol. scand.*, **25**, 49–76.

Fröhlich, A. & Loewi, O. (1910) Uber eine steigerung der adrenalinempfindlichkeit durch cocain. *Arch. exp. Path. Pharmak.*, **62**, 159–169.

Gillespie, J. S. (1973) Uptake of noradrenaline by smooth muscle. *Br. med. Bull.*, **29**, 136–141.

Hare, M. L. (1928) Tyramine oxidase. *Biochem. J.*, **22**, 968–979.

Iversen, L. L. (1965) The uptake of catecholamines at high perfusion concentrations in the rat isolated heart: a novel catecholamine uptake process. *Br. J. Pharmac.*, **25**, 18–33.

Langer, S. Z. (1977) Presynaptic receptors and their role in the regulation of transmitter release. *Br. J. Pharmac.*, **60**, 481–497.

Langley, J. N. (1905) On the reaction of cells and of nerve endings to certain poisons (nerve endings and receptive substance). *J. Physiol.*, **33**, 374–413.

Macmillan, W. H. (1959) A hypothesis concerning the effects of cocaine on the action of sympathomimetic amines. *Br. J. Pharmac.*, **14**, 385–391.

Oliver, G. & Schäffer, E. A. (1895) The physiological effects of extracts from the suprarenal capsules. *J. Physiol.*, **18**, 230–276.

Richter, D. (1937) Adrenaline and amine oxidase. *Biochem. J.*, **31**, 2022–2028.

Whitby, L. G., Axelrod, J. & Weil-Malherbe, H. (1961) The fate of H^3-norepinephrine in animals. *J. Pharmac. exp. Ther.*, **132**, 193–201.

GENERAL READING

Blaschko, H. (1973) Catecholamine Biosynthesis. *Br. med. Bull.*, **29**, 105–109.

Iversen, L. L. (1967) *The Uptake and Storage of Noradrenaline.* London: Cambridge University Press.

Iversen, L. L. (1973) Catecholamine uptake processes. *Br. med. Bull.*, **29**, 130–135.

Jenkinson, D. H. (1973) Classification and properties of peripheral adrenergic receptors. *Br. med. Bull.*, **29**, 142–147.

Sharman, D. F. (1973) The catabolism of catecholamines. *Br. med. Bull.*, **29**, 110–115.

Smith, A. D. (1973) Mechanisms involved in the release of noradrenaline from sympathetic nerves. *Br. med. Bull.*, **29**, 123–129.

Starke, K. (1977) Regulation of noradrenaline release by presynaptic receptor systems. *Rev. Physiol. Biochem. Pharmacol.*, **77**, 1–124.

9

Adrenoreceptor stimulants (sympathomimetics)

The discovery and role of noradrenaline as the transmitter substance released from most postganglionic sympathetic nerves was discussed in Chapter 3 and its synthesis, storage, release and inactivation in the body in Chapter 8. Many compounds structurally related to noradrenaline will similarly stimulate α and/or β-adrenoreceptors and a number of these compounds have been used clinically.

HISTORICAL NOTE ON THE DEVELOPMENT OF SYMPATHOMIMETIC SUBSTANCES

Barger & Dale (1910) were amongst the first workers to systematically examine the effects of a series of compounds with pharmacological actions resembling those of adrenaline; they suggested the term 'sympathomimetic' to describe the actions of these substances. Barger & Dale were mainly concerned with quantitative differences in the ability of the various compounds to raise the blood pressure of cats. However, arterial blood pressure is the resultant of a number of different parameters such as cardiac output, peripheral resistance and reflex modification of autonomic nerve activity all of which may be altered, sometimes in different ways, by various sympathomimetic substances. Thus pressor activity gives little indication of the mechanism of action of a compound. Nevertheless, in the past much has been written about the relative pressor potency of sympathomimetics, presumably because pressor activity is easily measured and because one of the main clinical uses for these substances is to raise systemic arterial blood pressure in hypotensive states. Later workers such as Tainter & Chang (1927) and Burn & Tainter (1931) demonstrated qualitative as well as quantitative differences between the actions of various sympathomimetic substances. They showed that chronic sympathectomy or cocaine pretreatment increased the responses of effector tissues to adrenaline but markedly reduced the responses of the related sympathomimetics ephedrine and tyramine. Qualitative differences between sympathomimetics were underlined by the discovery of Ahlquist (1948) of two distinct populations of adrenoreceptors possessing different structural requirements for activation. A further stimulus to interest in the mode of action of sympathomimetics was provided by the introduction into western medicine in the early 1950's of reserpine, a plant alkaloid which was shown by Bertler, Carlsson & Rosengren (1956) to deplete noradrenaline from sympathetic neurones by interfering with its intraneuronal storage. The classic experiments of Burn & Rand (1958) indicated that sympathomimetic substances could be broadly classified into two groups dependent on their activity on effector tissues pretreated with either cocaine or reserpine or in which the postganglionic sympathetic nerves had been sectioned and allowed to degenerate. The first group of sympathomimetics, which include noradrenaline and adrenaline, produce effects which are unaltered or increased by each of these treatments, whilst the second group, of which tyramine is the best known example, have their effects markedly reduced or abolished. The widely accepted interpretation of these observations is that the first group of substances produce their effects by direct activation of adrenoreceptors within effector tissues (*directly-acting sympathomimetics*) whilst the second group depend for their action on the existence of intact intraneuronal noradrenaline stores which they are believed to stochiometrically displace to produce their sympathomimetic effects (*indirectly-acting sympathomimetics*). Reserpine and chronic sympathectomy inhibit the actions of indirectly-acting sympathomimetics by removal of the neuronal noradrenaline stores whilst cocaine acts by preventing the uptake (by $Uptake_1$) of these substances into noradrenergic neurones and hence their ability to displace stored noradrenaline. The effects of directly-acting sympathomimetic amines are increased by sympathectomy and by cocaine pretreatment since both procedures inactivate the neuronal amine uptake mechanism ($Uptake_1$) and thus permit a higher concentration of the sympathomimetic to persist in the region of the adrenoreceptors in effector tissues. Reserpine does not inhibit $Uptake_1$ and therefore does not markedly alter the responses to directly-acting sympathomimetics. Reserpine is a particularly useful experimental tool for deciding on the mechanism of action of sympathomimetics since the depletion of neuronal noradrenaline which it produces can be partially reversed by the infusion of either noradrenaline or of one of its precursors which leads to a temporary restoration of the activity of indirectly-acting sympathomimetics (see Fig. 9.1).

The actions of sympathomimetic substances may therefore be complicated by differing activities in stimulating α- and β-adrenoreceptors and also in the relative components of direct and

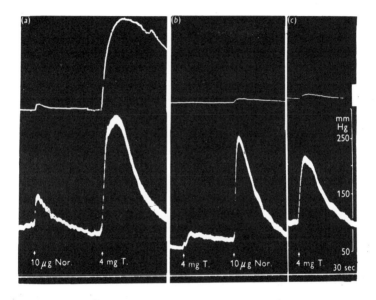

Fig. 9.1 Effect of reserpine on direct and indirectly-acting sympathomimetics in spinalised cats. Upper record contractions of the nictitating membrane; lower record arterial blood pressure. Responses in panel (a) are from a normal cat given intravenous injections of 10 μg noradrenaline (Nor) and 4 mg of tyramine (T). In the second panel is shown the much reduced response to the indirectly-acting tyramine and the undiminished response to the directly-acting noradrenaline in a cat depleted of neuronal noradrenaline by reserpine pretreatment. Between panels (b) and (c) noradrenaline (0·12 mg) was infused intravenously into the reserpine-treated cat and in (c) this has greatly increased the responses to tyramine (from Burn & Rand, 1958).

indirect activity. In practice α- and β-adrenoreceptor agonist activity and also direct and indirect effects form continuous spectra such that no substance is wholly specific for one type of action. Ephedrine is an example of a substance with mixed actions since it stimulates both α- and β-adrenoreceptors partly by direct stimulation of adrenoreceptors and partly indirectly by displacement of neuronal noradrenaline.

Structure-activity relationships of sympathomimetics

The parent compound of many sympathomimetic substances is phenylethylamine (more precisely β-phenylethylamine), the structure of which is shown in Fig. 9.2.

Phenylethylamine is itself a weak sympathomimetic substance with predominantly indirect effects. Its activity may be increased and/or modified by the substitution of groups on the aromatic ring, on the aliphatic side-chain or on the amine group.

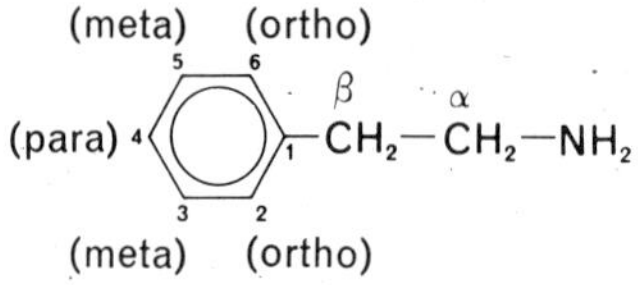

Fig. 9.2 Structure of phenylethylamine showing numbered and named positions on the benzene ring and indicating the α and β carbon atoms of the aliphatic side-chain.

Effects of adding hydroxyl groups to phenylethylamine

Addition of hydroxyl groups to the phenylethylamine structure increases the overall sympathomimetic activity of the molecule and produces qualitative changes in the type of activity. The important positions for hydroxylation are the 3 and 4 positions of the benzene ring and the β carbon atom (see Table 9.1). Hydroxylation of the 3-(meta) position on the ring is of more importance in increasing overall sympathomimetic activity than is hydroxylation of the 4-(para) position. Moreover, an hydroxyl group in the 3- position increases direct rather than indirect activity. Thus tyramine (4-hydroxyphenylethylamine) is of similar sympathomimetic potency to phenylethylamine but dopamine (3:4-dihydroxyphenylethylamine) is more potent than either and has a considerable direct component of activity. Phenylethylamine derivatives with hydroxyl groups in both 3 and 4 positions on the aromatic ring, such as dopamine and noradrenaline, may be considered to be derivatives of catechol and are therefore often called catecholamines. Addition of an hydroxyl group on the β-carbon atom of the aliphatic side-chain also increases sympathomimetic activity of the direct type. Thus noradrenaline, which has hydroxyl groups in positions 3 and 4 on the benzene ring and also one on the β-carbon atom, is a highly active sympathomimetic with virtually all its activity of the direct type.

Table 9.1 Effect of substituting hydroxyl groups onto the phenylethylamine molecule. Addition of one group in the 4-position (tyramine) has little or no effect on pressor potency or type of activity whilst addition of a further hydroxyl in the 3-position (dopamine) considerably increases pressor activity and introduces direct adrenoreceptor stimulant activity. Addition of a third hydroxyl group on the β-carbon atom causes a further marked increase in pressor potency and the activity is almost entirely due to direct stimulation of adrenoreceptors.

sympathomimetic substance	pressor activity	type of activity
$\langle\bigcirc\rangle$—CH$_2$—CH$_2$—NH$_2$ phenylethylamine	weak	indirect
HO—$\langle\bigcirc\rangle$—CH$_2$—CH$_2$—NH$_2$ tyramine	unaffected or slightly increased	indirect
HO—$\langle\bigcirc\rangle$—CH$_2$—CH$_2$—NH$_2$ (HO) dopamine	considerably increased	direct and indirect
HO—$\langle\bigcirc\rangle$—CH—CH$_2$—NH$_2$ (HO) OH noradrenaline	markedly increased	direct

Effect of substitution on the amine group of phenylethylamine

Addition of alkyl groups to the amine group of phenylethylamine increases β and reduces α-adrenoreceptor stimulant activity. This type of substitution is of most consequence in those compounds, such as the catecholamines, which have marked direct sympathomimetic effects. The effect of alkyl group addition to the amine group of noradrenaline is shown in Table 9.2. Addition of a methyl group, to give adrenaline, increases β but does not markedly change α-adrenoreceptor potency whilst an N-isopropyl group produces a compound (isoprenaline) with marked β but little α-adrenoreceptor agonist activity.

Modifications of the phenylethylamine structure producing changes in the metabolism/inactivation of the molecule

Substitution at some sites on the phenylethylamine molecule produces marked changes in its rate of inactivation and hence

Table 9.2 Effect of N-substitution on the adrenoreceptor stimulant activity of noradrenaline. Addition of a methyl group to the terminal nitrogen atom (adrenaline) conveys considerable β-adrenoreceptor stimulant potency whilst addition of an isopropyl group (isoprenaline) further increases β-, but practically removes α-, adrenoreceptor stimulant activity.

sympathomimetic substance	adrenoreceptor stimulant activity
HO—⟨benzene ring, HO—⟩—CH(OH)—CH$_2$—NH$_2$ noradrenaline	mainly α
HO—⟨benzene ring, HO—⟩—CH(OH)—CH$_2$—NH—CH$_3$ adrenaline (N-methylnoradrenaline)	α and β
HO—⟨benzene ring, HO—⟩—CH(OH)—CH$_2$—NH·CH(CH$_3$)$_2$ isoprenaline (N-isopropylnoradrenaline)	mainly β

duration of action. Prolongation of the duration of action of a sympathomimetic substance may produce qualitative as well as quantitative changes in its activity since it may gain access to sites which it would not otherwise have done. Sympathomimetics are inactivated in the body by various mechanisms which include those used to inactivate the naturally occurring catecholamines. Thus sympathomimetics may be oxidatively deaminated by monoamine oxidase, O-methylated by catechol-O-methyltransferase and/or taken up (by Uptake$_1$) into noradrenergic neurones. Phenylethylamine is metabolized almost entirely by monoamine oxidase since it has no hydroxyl group in the 3-position on the ring for methylation by catechol-O-methyltransferase nor is it a good substrate for Uptake$_1$. Phenylethylamine and its derivatives may be rendered immune to the action of monoamine oxidase by addition of a methyl group to the α-carbon atom which effectively protects the amine group from oxidation. α-Methylphenylethylamine (amphetamine) has similar indirect sympathomimetic activity to phenylethylamine but because of its persistence in the body it is able to penetrate into the central nervous system where it causes stimulant and other effects which have been utilised clinically.

Catechol-O-methyltransferase will attack those phenylethylamine derivatives having an hydroxyl group in the 3-(meta) position on the benzene ring. Since this hydroxyl group is important for direct adrenoreceptor stimulant potency it is difficult to modify it without loss of activity. However, salbutamol (see later) is a clinically-useful sympathomimetic substance in which this group has been chemically modified to prevent destruction by catechol-O-methyltransferase. Many sympathomimetics are to some extent transported into noradrenergic neurones by Uptake$_1$ and this includes most phenylethylamine derivatives having at least one hydroxyl group on the benzene ring. Some of these substances, such as metaraminol, may displace noradrenaline from its intraneuronal storage sites and/or may inhibit Uptake$_1$ leading to changes in the effectiveness of activating sympathetic nerves and also in the actions of other sympathomimetic substances.

THE NATURE OF ADRENORECEPTORS

As with other types of receptor much is written, but little known, concerning the structure and functioning of adrenoreceptors. Belleau (1963) has proposed that the receptor for catecholamines is a single structure with α and β sites (see Fig. 9.3). At physiological pH the catecholamines exist in an ionic form with a positively charged nitrogen atom. According to Belleau β effects are favoured by combination of the catechol hydroxyl groups to the β site of the receptor via formation of a metal ion complex. Combination of the positively charged nitrogen atom of the catecholamine with a negatively charged group (possibly phosphate) on the receptor favours α-effects. It follows that substitution on the nitrogen atom with bulky groups such as isopropyl (as in isoprenaline) interferes with attachment to the α site and therefore favours β-effects through combination of the catechol hydroxyl groups. It is suggested that when both sites are occupied then α-effects are produced whilst combination through the catechol hydroxyl groups alone favours β-effects. Kunos & Nickerson (1976) have provided evidence which is consistent with Belleau's view of a single adrenoreceptor with different sites modulating α and β effects. They found that in the frog heart increases in force of contraction produced by adrenaline were abolished by α-adrenoreceptor blockers at temperatures below 17 °C and by β-adrenoreceptor blockers when the temperature was raised to 23 °C or above. They suggested that α and β-adrenoreceptors may be different allosteric forms of the same basic structure.

It has been suggested that β effects are mediated by formation of cyclic AMP in effector cells and that the β-adrenoreceptor may be localised on the enzyme adenyl cyclase which catalyses the breakdown of ATP to cyclic AMP. The main objection to this

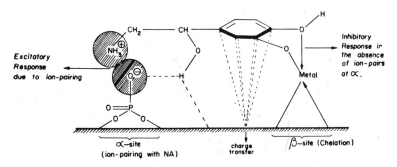

Fig. 9.3 Belleau's (1963) concept of a single adrenoreceptor mediating both α and β effects. Formation of an ionic bond between the positively charged nitrogen atom of noradrenaline and a negatively charged phosphate group on the receptor favours α-effects whilst β-effects result from combination of the ring hydroxyl groups of noradrenaline with the β-site of the receptor via a metal ion chelate and in the absence of an ionic bond at the α-site.

theory stems from the rapidity of onset of β effects after administration of β-adrenoreceptor stimulants which occur before any detectable change in cyclic AMP levels.

No model or hypothesis thus far advanced to explain the nature of adrenoreceptors satisfactorily explains all of the available experimental data. Basic questions remain unanswered. For instance, why does the body utilise noradrenaline as the neurotransmitter substance in the sympathetic nerves supplying the heart (where the adrenoreceptors are predominantly of the β type) as well as the vasomotor nerves supplying blood vessels of the skin (where the receptors are mainly of the α type)? It is difficult to imagine how noradrenaline can function efficiently at both sites whereas a β-adrenoreceptor stimulant such as isoprenaline only produces effects on the heart. It may be that neurotransmitter substances are able to induce conformational changes either in themselves or in the adrenoreceptors which are not readily mimicked by other substances.

General pharmacological actions of sympathomimetics
Innes & Nickerson (1975) in reviewing the actions of sympathomimetics considered that their effects could be classified into
five broad groups:
1. Peripheral excitatory actions such as those on smooth muscle
of blood vessels in the skin and the smooth muscle of the splenic
capsule;
2. Peripheral inhibitory actions on some smooth muscle such as
that of the respiratory and gastrointestinal tracts and of blood
vessels supplying skeletal muscle;
3. A cardiac excitatory action causing an increase in force and/or
rate of cardiac contraction;
4. Metabolic actions such as an increase in rate of glycogenolysis
in liver and muscle and liberation of free fatty acids from adipose
tissue;
5. Central nervous system excitatory effects such as stimulation
of respiration and, with some agents, euphoria and increased
wakefulness. Individual sympathomimetic substances do not
exhibit all of these actions to a similar extent and their specificity
for one or more types of action is generally the basis for the use of
these drugs in various clinical conditions. The widest spectrum of
sympathomimetic activity is probably exhibited by the naturally
occurring catecholamine adrenaline since it is a potent stimulant
of the two main adrenoreceptor types (α and β) which mediate
the majority of sympathomimetic actions.

CLINICAL USES FOR SYMPATHOMIMETICS

The main clinical uses for the sympathomimetics are based on
their actions on the cardiovascular and respiratory system.

Cardiovascular system
substances which stimulate the α-adrenoreceptors in resistance
vessels induce an increase in peripheral resistance which often
produces an increase in the level of systemic arterial blood pressure. For this reason many sympathomimetics have been used to
raise the arterial blood pressure in hypotensive states occurring
for instance after traumatic or surgical shock or as a result of
myocardial infarction. All of these conditions carry a high risk of
mortality and the usefulness or otherwise of pressor substances
in aiding recovery has been very difficult to assess and remains
an area of considerable debate and controversy. In particular the

value of raising arterial blood pressure in hypotensive states has been questioned since higher blood pressure is no guarantee of increased blood perfusion of vital tissues such as the brain, heart and kidneys, and some sympathomimetics may even further reduce blood perfusion of some organs by virtue of their vaso-constrictor action. Certainly the use of vasoconstrictor drugs in hypovolaemic states is illogical unless steps have been taken to restore circulatory volume by infusion of whole blood, plasma or a suitable plasma expander. Similarly, some sympathomimetics which have been used to treat circulatory collapse have marked stimulant effects on the myocardium and may increase cardiac output. However, some of these substances, of which adrenaline is an example, also caused marked increases in myocardial oxygen usage which may lead to an overall reduction in the efficiency of the heart especially if the myocardium is already damaged. Some of the more recently introduced sympatho-mimetics such as dopamine (see later) produce only mild cardiac stimulation and little effect on systemic arterial blood pressure and may increase blood flow in some important vascular beds such as that of the kidneys. The basic underlying cardiovascular defects occurring in various hypotensive states remain poorly understood which adds a further difficulty to the proper eval-uation of drugs used in cardiovascular support.

Other uses of sympathomimetics based on their effects on blood vessels includes their use by local application to reduce bleeding from superficial wounds, to prevent the undue spread and absorption of local anaesthetics and to cause vasoconstriction of the nasal mucosa in cases of nasal stuffiness resulting from allergic conditions or common colds.

Respiratory system

Sympathomimetics which stimulate β-adrenoreceptors are used to relax the bronchial smooth muscle in conditions such as asthma. With substances such as isoprenaline and adrenaline the bronchodilator effect is accompanied by marked cardiac stim-ulation. However, derivatives of isoprenaline such as isoetharine and salbutamol have been developed which stimulate preferent-ially the β-adrenoreceptors of the respiratory tract whilst producing little effect on those of the heart. This observation led Lands and his colleagues (1967) to suggest a sub-classification of β-adrenoreceptors; he called the receptors in the heart and small intestine β_1 and those in the bronchi, vascular beds and uterus β_2.

Some sympathomimetics such as dexamphetamine were formerly much used for their stimulant effects on the brain. These effects include feelings of well-being (*euphoria*), increased wakefulness, an improved attitude to uninteresting or repetitive work and a suppression of appetite for food (*anorexia*). The widespread use of these drugs both by patients who had been prescribed them them and by others such as athletes who prized their central stimulant effects, led to a considerable abuse problem. The pendulum of public and scientific opinion has now swung heavily against these drugs and they are at present little used clinically but their illicit use remains a problem. There are other minor uses for sympathomimetics such as to produce mydriasis and to relax the uterus in dysmenorhoea and in premature labour and these will be mentioned under the individual agents.

A very considerable number of sympathomimetic substances are at present in clinical use and many more have been tried in the past. The actions and uses of the three catecholamines noradrenaline, adrenaline and isoprenaline will be described first in some detail since these substances cover almost the entire spectrum of actions and uses of the other sympathomimetics which are used clinically for their peripheral effects. Other sympathomimetics in common clinical usage will be described in groups classified according to their main clinical use.

SYMPATHOMIMETICS IN CLINICAL USE

The catecholamines noradrenaline, adrenaline and isoprenaline

Noradrenaline

$$HO-\underset{\underset{HO}{\displaystyle|}}{\bigcirc}-CH-CH_2-NH_2$$
$$\qquad\qquad\overset{|}{OH}$$

$(-)$-Noradrenaline is the transmitter substance released from noradrenergic sympathetic nerves and its effects in the body in most respects resemble the effects of sympathetic activation. It is the $(-)$-isomer of noradrenaline which is used clinically; in the USA it is known as *levarterenol* or *norepinephrine*. The basis for the clinical use of noradrenaline is it's ability to raise systemic arterial blood pressure by causing vasoconstriction resulting from its α-adrenoreceptor stimulant activity. It is ineffective by mouth due to rapid destruction in the gastrointestinal tract but when administered by injection it raises both systolic and diastolic systemic arterial pressures (see Fig. 9.4). The pressor response to noradrenaline is due almost entirely to increased peripheral resistance as a result of vasoconstriction, cardiac output is usually little affected. In most subjects usual clinical

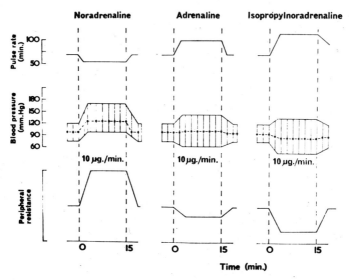

Fig. 9.4 Effect on pulse rate, blood pressure and peripheral resistance of intravenous infusions of noradrenaline, adrenaline and isoprenaline (isopropylnoradrenaline) in man. (From Allwood, Cobbold & Ginsburg, 1963).

doses of noradrenaline produce bradycardia which results from activation of the baroreceptor reflexes leading to increased vagal (inhibitory) and decreased sympathetic (excitatory) influences on the heart. In patients with markedly reduced cardiac output noradrenaline may increase it by causing increased venous return as a result of venoconstriction. Cardiac oxygen consumption is increased by noradrenaline even in the absence of changes in cardiac output. This is due to the increase in cardiac work required to maintain cardiac output in the presence of an increased peripheral resistance.

Noradrenaline decreases blood flow to the kidneys, brain, liver, and usually also to skeletal muscle, but markedly increases blood flow to the myocardium by producing coronary vasodilatation. The mechanism of the coronary dilatation produced by noradrenaline and by many other sympathomimetics is complex, the main factors involved being increased flow due to raised arterial pressure and production by the myocardium of vaso-dilator metabolites, such as adenosine, which result from the increased myocardial energy usage.

The other sympathomimetic actions of noradrenaline such as increasing blood sugar level and effects on the central nervous system are not prominent in man at the usual therapeutic dose levels.

Clinical uses and dosage. Noradrenaline is used clinically as the bitartrate (Noradrenaline Acid Tartrate BP) which contains approximately 50 per cent of noradrenaline base. It is usually administered by slow intravenous infusion at a dose level of 2 to 20 micrograms per minute of base to raise blood pressure in certain hypotensive states such as those occurring after surgical removal of a phaeochromocytoma, resulting from overdosage with hypotensive agents, surgical shock or myocardial infarction. It is usually administered in a solution containing about 8 micrograms per ml of noradrenaline bitartrate dissolved in Sodium Chloride and Dextrose Solution BP or in Dextrose Injection BP.

Intravenous injections of noradrenaline produce only brief increases in blood pressure due to rapid destruction in the bloodstream by catechol-O-methyltransferase, uptake by nor-adrenergic neurones and to a lesser extent to destruction by monoamine oxidase. However, when administered by slow intravenous infusion noradrenaline can be used to stabilize the blood pressure at any desired level and infusions may be main-tained continuously for several days. Long-term infusions may lead to some loss of responsiveness to noradrenaline which may necessitate increases in the dose administered. Infusions need to be discontinued gradually otherwise precipitous falls in pressure, similar to that often seen after removal of a phaeochromocytoma may occur. The reason for this fall in blood pressure after noradrenaline infusions is not entirely clear but may be related to both desensitisation of vascular α-adrenoreceptors to nor-adrenaline and also to a reflex reduction in sympathetic nerve traffic. There are other complications associated with the use of noradrenaline to raise blood pressure; the bitartrate salt is strongly acidic and accidental leakage from the site of infusion may cause severe necrosis of surrounding tissues. The pressor activity of noradrenaline may be greatly increased in patients concurrently receiving drugs, such as tricyclic antidepressants or noradrenergic neurone blockers, which inhibit the neuronal amine uptake mechanism (Uptake$_1$).

Noradrenaline solutions containing 10 to 20 micrograms per ml of base are occasionally mixed with injections of local anaesthetics to limit their spread and absorption and solutions containing about 200 micrograms per ml have been used by topical application to control capillary bleeding.

A convenient preparation of noradrenaline is Strong Sterile Noradrenaline Solution BPC which contains the equivalent of 1 mg/ml of noradrenaline base. This solution is too strong for direct injection but is used to prepare more dilute solutions for intravenous infusion immediately prior to use. Noradrenaline Injection BPC contains 4 micrograms per ml noradrenaline base dissolved in Sodium Chloride and Dextrose Solution BP or in Dextrose Injection BP. Noradrenaline bitartrate is available commercially in ampoules containing the equivalent of either 1 mg/ml noradrenaline base (LEVOPHED) or 100 micrograms per ml (LEVOPHED SPECIAL SOLUTION); the latter solution is intended for direct intravenous or intracardiac injection for use in cardiac resuscitation.

Adrenaline

$$HO-\!\!\!\!\!\!\bigcirc\!\!\!\!\!\!-CH-CH_2-NH-CH_3$$

The clinically used form of adrenaline is the naturally-occurring $(-)$-isomer which in the USA is known as *epinephrine*. The presence of a methyl substituent on the amine group of the molecule confers marked β-adrenoreceptor stimulant potency on adrenaline whilst its α-potency is at least as great as that of noradrenaline. The clinical uses of adrenaline are based on both α and β-adrenoreceptor stimulant potency. Its most important effects are those on the cardiovascular and respiratory systems and its metabolic actions.

Cardiovascular system
The cardiovascular effects produced in man by an intravenous infusion of adrenaline are shown in Fig. 9.4. Systolic pressure is raised whilst diastolic pressure is lowered and mean pressure little changed. Heart rate is increased and overall peripheral resistance is reduced. The differences in the cardiovascular effects of adrenaline and noradrenaline are accountable in terms

of the β-effects of adrenaline. The increase in systolic pressure caused by adrenaline is due entirely to increased cardiac output resulting from cardiac β-adrenoreceptor stimulation which evokes increases in both cardiac contractile force and rate. Adrenaline causes a mixture of vasoconstriction and vasodilatation in different vascular beds depending on the relative proportions of α and β receptors present. Thus vasoconstriction occurs in the blood vessels of the skin, mucosa and kidney which contain mainly α-adrenoreceptors whilst the vasculature of skeletal muscles, which contain mainly β-adrenoreceptors, are dilated. The overall effect is a reduction in peripheral resistance which leads to a drop in diastolic pressure. Cardiac output may also be elevated by adrenaline because of the increased venous return which it causes resulting from venoconstriction. Adrenaline, like noradrenaline, causes a marked increase in coronary blood flow but since its cardiac stimulant effects are much greater the increased myocardial oxygen usage which it promotes may produce a greater reduction in myocardial efficiency than is produced by noradrenaline. The cardiovascular effects of adrenaline are to some extent dependent on the dose and rate of administration. For instance, rapid intravenous injection of a moderate dose may cause an increase in diastolic as well as systolic pressure and may induce a reflex bradycardia. Adrenaline, particularly if administered by the intravenous route, carries a considerable risk of inducing cardiac arrhythmias due to its effects in producing an over-excitable state of the cardiac muscle cells.

Respiratory system
Adrenaline has a brief and unimportant respiratory stimulant action but it produces important consequences for respiration in cases of bronchospasm because of its β action in relaxing bronchial smooth muscle. It is likely also that the α-adrenoreceptor stimulant activity of adrenaline is of importance when the drug is used to treat asthma since it relieves congestion of the bronchial mucosa by causing vasoconstriction.

Metabolic effects
Adrenaline increases blood glucose levels by a mechanism which involves the formation of cyclic-AMP (from ATP) by activation of the enzyme adenyl cyclase. Cyclic-AMP in turn stimulates a phosphorylase enzyme which catalyses the breakdown of glycogen in liver and muscle firstly to glucose-1-phosphate and

eventually to glucose in liver cells and lactic acid in muscle cells. This glycogenolytic action of adrenaline is thought to be mediated via β-adrenoreceptors. Adrenaline also has a hyperglycaemic action by suppressing insulin secretion via a mechanism involving α-adrenoreceptor stimulation.

Adrenaline raises the plasma level of free fatty acids by activating a lipase which accelerates the breakdown of triglycerides. The lipolytic action of adrenaline is also mediated via cyclic-AMP and β-adrenoreceptors. The overall stimulation of metabolism in man produced by conventional doses of adrenaline produces an increase in the order of 20 to 30 per cent in oxygen consumption.

Clinical uses and dosage. Adrenaline BP is the base; it is most often used clinically in the form of the bitartrate salt (Adrenaline Acid Tartrate BP) which contains approximately 1 mg of adrenaline in every 1·8 mg of salt.

Adrenaline, like noradrenaline, is ineffective orally and is most often used by the subcutaneous route. Adrenaline Injection (BP, BNF) contains the equivalent of 1 mg/ml of adrenaline base dissolved in Water for Injections BP. In acute bronchial asthma the adult subcutaneous dose is 0·2 to 0·5 mg but in status asthmaticus up to 0·5 mg may be injected subcutaneously on up to three occasions at 10 minutely intervals to abort the attack. Adrenaline is also available commercially as a constituent of spray solutions and aerosol preparations intended for inhalation. The aerosol preparations deliver a metered dose of either 250 micrograms (PRESSURISED BROVON) or 280 micrograms (MEDIHALER-EPI) of adrenaline.

Adrenaline has been widely used in the symptomatic treatment of allergic conditions such as urticaria, allergic eczema, serum and X-ray sickness and allergic shock. In all of these conditions it is administered subcutaneously in adult doses up to 1 mg and it relieves the itching, pain, swelling and oedema associated with these conditions.

The uses of adrenaline for treating conditions of the cardiovascular system are limited because it has a marked tendency to cause cardiac arrhthymias including ventricular fibrillation which may be rapidly fatal. The arrhthymic actions of adrenaline are markedly potentiated in the presence of some general anaesthetics such as chloroform and cyclopropane and to a lesser extent by halothane and trichloroethylene. It has been used (0·6 mg subcutaneously) to treat heart-block associated with syncope (Stokes-Adams attacks) and also by direct intracardiac injection (0·25 mg) in cardiac emergencies arising during surgery. Adrenaline has in the past been used intravenously to treat circulatory collapse but it is now generally considered to be too hazardous by this route. In concentrations ranging from 20 micrograms per ml to 1 mg/ml adrenaline solutions are used by local application to check capillary bleeding. It is particularly useful for this purpose in dentistry after tooth extraction and in surgery of the eye, ear, nose and throat.

Adrenaline solutions are used in ophthalmology for instillation into the eye to treat conjunctival congestion and to control haemorrhages and to reduce intraocular pressure in cases of simple glaucoma. The effectiveness of adrenaline in the treatment of glaucoma is believed to be due to the reduction in the rate of production of aqueous humour which it produces. Neutral Adrenaline Eye-Drops (BPC, BNF) contain 1 per cent w/v adrenaline dissolved in borate buffer; a similar preparation is available commercially (EPPY).

Adrenaline has a reputation for being effective in the form of cream when massaged into skin in the treatment of fibrositis. Proprietary products are available which contain 1 in 5000 of adrenaline in a cream base but there is no evidence to suggest that they are more effective than massage alone.

Isoprenaline

Isoprenaline is a synthetic catecholamine derived from noradrenaline by substitution of an isopropyl group on the nitrogen atom of the aliphatic side-chain. The commercially available form is the racemate; it is known as *isoproterenol* in the USA. The pharmacological actions of isoprenaline are almost entirely due to its powerful β-adrenoreceptor stimulant activity; it is almost without effect on α-adrenoreceptors. The effects of an intravenous infusion of isoprenaline on the cardiovascular system of man are shown in Fig. 9.4. Its main cardiovascular effects are a marked increase in cardiac output, as a result of stimulation of cardiac β-adrenoreceptors subserving increases in rate and force of the heart beat, associated with a reduction in peripheral resistance due to vasodilatation especially of the blood vessels of skeletal muscles. In usual therapeutic doses (as in Fig. 9.4) isoprenaline may slightly raise systolic blood pressure because of cardiac stimulation whilst diastolic pressure is lowered due to the fall in peripheral resistance. Isoprenaline increases coronary blood flow and stimulates myocardial oxygen usage. Intravenous doses of isoprenaline of the order of 1 microgram per kg produce in man a marked lowering of both systolic and diastolic pressures.

Isoprenaline, like adrenaline, has potent metabolic effects in man; it causes less hyperglycaemia than adrenaline probably because it releases insulin by stimulating β-adrenoreceptors in the pancreatic islet cells. However, it is as effective as adrenaline in raising plasma free fatty acid levels. Other effects of β-adrenoreceptor stimulation such as inhibition of the gastro-intestinal tract and stimulation of the central nervous system are not prominent with therapeutic dose levels. The most important action of isoprenaline from the clinical standpoint is its effect in stimulating β-adrenoreceptors in the respiratory tract leading to bronchodilatation and a reduction in airways resistance.

Isoprenaline is somewhat erratically absorbed when taken orally but absorption is more regular and complete if the tablets are allowed to slowly dissolve under the tongue (*sublingual administration*). The reason for this difference is that after absorption from the small intestine isoprenaline is rapidly inactivated in the liver whereas absorption through the buccal mucous membrane enables it to enter the general circulation before reaching the liver. Isoprenaline is very well absorbed after either parenteral administration or inhalation. The metabolism of isoprenaline is to some extent determined by the route of administration; after oral administration it is mainly conjugated in the liver whilst after intravenous injection it is mainly methylated by catechol-O-methyltransferase.

Clinical uses and dosage. The most used form of isoprenaline is Isoprenaline Sulphate BP which is used in the form of tablets at an adult dose of 10 to 20 mg sublingually three times daily. Relief of bronchospasm after sublingual administration usually commences after 2 to 4 minutes. Isoprenaline Tablets BP each contain 10 mg of isoprenaline sulphate. More rapid relief may be obtained by inhaling the drug in a finely powdered form administered by means of a pressurised aerosol. Two aerosol preparations containing isoprenaline sulphate receive official (BPC) recognition; Isoprenaline Aerosol Inhalation BPC delivers metered doses of 80 micrograms of isoprenaline sulphate and Strong Isoprenaline Aerosol Inhalation BPC 400 microgram doses. The maximal single recommended dose of isoprenaline sulphate by inhalation is 1·2 mg with a maximum of 3·2 mg in any 24 hour period.

Isoprenaline, like adrenaline, may cause cardiac hyper-excitability and fatal arrhthymias have resulted from its excessive usage particularly in the form of aerosols. In the mid-1960's it was noticed that the number of sudden unexpected deaths amongst asthmatic patients was rising quite steeply. The increase in deaths was highest in children and young persons up to 20 years of age and appeared to be associated with excessive use of isoprenaline-containing aerosol preparations. The precise cause of these deaths has not been determined but the evidence from animal studies suggests that the tendency of isoprenaline to cause cardiac arrhthymias is much more pronounced during periods of hypoxia and/or cardiac overload such as may occur during severe asthmatic attacks. It has also been suggested, but not proved, that the propellant substances used in the aerosols may have deleterious effects on the myocardium when used in high doses. The apparent greater toxicity of the aerosol preparations over tablets may be simply due to the greater ease with which repeated doses may be administered by aerosol coupled with ignorance, at the time, of any likely untoward reactions from taking repeated doses. Since early 1967 there has been a sharp fall in deaths from asthma which has been paralleled by a reduction in the use of aerosol preparations containing isoprenaline.

Isoprenaline is occasionally used by the oral or intravenous route to treat heart block and the hydrochloride salt (Isoprenaline Hydrochloride BPC) is used in these preparations. For the oral treatment of heart block isoprenaline hydrochloride in the form of slow release tablets each containing 30 mg are used (Isoprenaline Slow Tablets, BNF; proprietary preparation SAVENTRINE TABLETS) with a maximal daily dose of 750 mg. Isoprenaline hydrochloride is also available as an injection for intravenous use containing 2 mg of isoprenaline hydrochloride in a 2 ml aqueous solution which is further diluted before use. Dilute solutions of isoprenaline hydrochloride (20 to 40 micrograms per ml have been used intravenously to treat heart block and to provide cardiovascular support in some hypotensive states.

Isoprenaline is a constituent of a large number of proprietary preparations mostly designed for use in the treatment of asthma. However, with the clear evidence of cardiac toxicity which it may cause and with the emergence of other β-adrenoreceptor stimulants having much more specific effects for β-adreno-receptors of the respiratory tract it is likely that the use of these preparations will decline in the future.

SYMPATHOMIMETIC SUBSTANCES USED MAINLY IN HYPOTENSIVE STATES

The structures of most of the substances commonly used in the United Kingdom to raise blood pressure in hypotensive states are shown in Table 9.3.

Phenylephrine Hydrochloride

This substance differs from adrenaline only in lacking the hydroxy group in the 4-(para) position on the benzene ring. It is less potent in raising blood pressure than noradrenaline but has a more prolonged action. Its actions are due mainly to direct stimulation of α-adrenoreceptors; it has only very weak stimulant effects on β-adrenoreceptors. It raises blood pressure almost entirely by increasing peripheral resistance, cardiac

Table 9.3 Structural formulae of sympathomimetics used mainly to raise arterial blood pressure.

Structural formula	name(s)
$\text{HO}-\langle\text{ring}\rangle-\text{CH(OH)}-\text{CH}_2-\text{NH}-\text{CH}_3$	phenylephrine
$\text{HO}-\langle\text{ring}\rangle-\text{CH(OH)}-\text{CH}_2-\text{NH}-\text{CH}_3$	oxedrine (SYMPATOL)
$\text{HO}-\langle\text{ring}\rangle-\text{CH(OH)}-\text{CH(CH}_3)-\text{NH}_2$	metaraminol (ARAMINE)
$\text{CH}_3\text{O}-\langle\text{ring}\rangle(\text{CH}_3\text{O})-\text{CH(OH)}-\text{CH(CH}_3)-\text{NH}_2$	methoxamine
$\langle\text{ring}\rangle-\text{CH}_2-\text{C(CH}_3)_2-\text{NH}-\text{CH}_3$	mephentermine

output being little affected. It produces a reflex slowing of the heart due to its peripheral vasoconstrictor activity. It dilates the coronary vessels. It is metabolised in the body by monoamine oxidase and probably also by catechol-O-methyltransferase.

Clinical uses and dosage. In the treatment of hypotensive states phenylephrine may be used by intramuscular, subcutaneous or intravenous routes. By subcutaneous or intramuscular routes it is administered in a usual dose of 5 mg followed by further doses of 10 mg as necessary. By the intravenous route doses up to 20 mg may be administered by slow infusion when diluted with a suitable intravenous fluid to give a concentration of 10 to 40 micrograms per ml of phenylephrine. It may be administered by rapid intravenous injection in doses up to 0·5 mg to induce reflex bradycardia which may restore normal cardiac rhythm in patients suffering from paroxysmal auricular tachycardia. Phenylephrine is less likely than adrenaline and noradrenaline to induce cardiac arrhthymias even in patients anaesthetised with the anaesthetics chloroform, cyclopropane or halothane which are particularly likely to give rise to arrhthymias in the presence of adrenaline.

The drug is irregularly absorbed orally but it has been administered by this route in adult doses up to 150 mg daily to treat orthostatic hypotension and up to 75 mg daily in allergic conditions and nasal congestion. Phenylephrine, like adrenaline, is used for most of the peripheral actions for which sympathomimetics have been utilised. Thus solutions containing 0·5 mg/ml have been used to prevent the spread of local anaesthetics and it is commonly used in 0·25 to 0·5 per cent solutions to produce local vasoconstriction in nasal congestion. Solutions containing up to 10 per cent of phenylephrine hydrochloride are used in ophthalmology to produce mydriasis without accompanying cycloplegia.

Phenylephrine Injection BP contains 10 mg/ml of the drug and is used undiluted for intramuscular or subcutaneous use and diluted with a suitable intravenous fluid for intravenous use. The official (BPC, BNF) eye drops contain 100 mg/ml phenylephrine hydrochloride. The drug is a constituent of a number of proprietary preparations, most of which are intended to produce nasal decongestion.

Oxedrine Tartrate
This substance differs from phenylephrine only in the position of the hydroxy group on the benzene ring. It is considerably less

potent than phenylephrine but its actions are qualitatively similar.

Clinical uses and dosage. Oxedrine is used to treat hypotension either by the oral route (maximum dose 150 mg daily) or by subcutaneous or intramuscular injection (dose up to 100 mg). It is available as a liquid preparation containing 10 per cent oxedrine tartrate for oral use and as an injection containing 60 mg/ml. The proprietary name is SYMPATOL.

Metaraminol Tartrate

This substance produces circulatory effects which resemble those of noradrenaline but are more prolonged since it is immune to destruction by monoamine oxidase because of the presence of a methyl substituent on the α-carbon atom. Its sympathomimetic effects are partly mediated by direct stimulation of α-adrenoreceptors and partly due to indirect release of noradrenaline from noradrenergic neurones. It raises blood pressure mainly by increasing peripheral resistance and has little effect on cardiac output unless this is depressed. In patients with a very low cardiac output or in whom reflex bradycardia is abolished by atropine metaraminol may increase cardiac output showing that it probably has some stimulant activity on cardiac β-adrenoreceptors.

Clinical uses and dosage. Metaraminol is used in hypotensive states in doses of 2 to 10 mg by subcutaneous or intramuscular injection. It is sometimes given by slow intravenous infusion in a concentration of 30 to 200 micrograms per ml in Dextrose or Sodium Chloride Injection. In a hypotensive crisis up to 5 mg may be given by rapid intravenous injection.

Metaraminol Injection BP contains 10 mg/ml of metaraminol tartrate either in 1 ml ampoules or in a 10 ml multi-dose vial. It is available in the same forms under the proprietary name of ARAMINE.

Methoxamine Hydrochloride

This substance raises both systolic and diastolic arterial pressures and the effects of a single parenteral dose may persist for up to 90 minutes. Its pressor effect is due to the increase in peripheral resistance which it causes by direct stimulation of α-adrenoreceptors in blood vessels. Cardiac rate is reflexly slowed and cardiac output little affected. The drug has been reported to block cardiac β-adrenoreceptors and thus no stimulation of cardiac rate occurs even when reflex effects on the heart are abolished. The β-adrenoreceptor blocking action of the drug may be the reason why it does not cause cardiac arrhthymias in clinical use. Its prolonged action is due to the fact that it is not destroyed in the body by either monoamine oxidase or catechol-O-methyltransferase.

Clinical uses and dosage. In hypotensive states the drug is usually administered intramuscularly in doses of 5 to 20 mg. In emergencies 5 to 10 mg may be injected intravenously at a rate of about 1 mg per minute. Methoxamine Injection BPC, BNF contains 20 mg/ml of the drug.

A solution containing 0·25 per cent is used as a nasal decongestant (proprietary name VASYLOX).

Mephentermine Sulphate

This substance is another example of a sympathomimetic not readily metabolised in the body and thus having a very prolonged duration of action. The sympathomimetic effects of mephentermine are mediated almost entirely indirectly through neuronal noradrenaline release which acts upon both α and β-adrenoreceptors. The rise in blood pressure which it causes is thus due to increases in both cardiac output and peripheral resistance. The effect on heart rate is variable and dependent to some extent on the degree of vagal tone; coronary blood flow is increased.

Clinical uses and dosage. To treat hypotension mephentermine may be injected intramuscularly in doses of 15 to 30 mg which produces effects lasting up to 2 hours. When used intravenously it is either injected in doses of 15 to 60 mg over 1 to 2 minutes or is slowly infused after dilution with a suitable intravenous fluid to give a concentration of 0·3 to 1·2 mg/ml of mephentermine. Mephentermine Injection BP contains 15 mg/ml of mephentermine sulphate.

Dopamine Hydrochloride

Dopamine is the naturally occurring catecholamine which is the immediate precursor in the body of noradrenaline and which additionally has a neurotransmitter function in its own right in the mammalian central nervous system and possibly also in some peripheral tissues. Dopamine hydrochloride has recently been introduced into therapy for the treatment of shock syndromes associated with reduced cardiac output and blood pressure. It is ineffective orally but intravenous infusions of usual human doses cause an increase in cardiac output with little effect on cardiac rate. Overall peripheral resistance is lowered; systolic pressure is slightly elevated and diastolic pressure lowered. Dopamine causes a marked dilatation of the mesenteric and renal vascular beds. Most of the cardiovascular effects of dopamine are produced by virtue of its stimulant effects on both α and β-adrenoreceptors. However, its effects on the renal and mesenteric vasculatures are thought to be mediated by stimulation of specific dopamine receptors.

The potential advantages of dopamine over other sympathomimetics used for cardiovascular support are:
1. It causes cardiac stimulation with little increase in myocardial oxygen consumption;
2. It appears less likely to cause cardiac arrhthymias than some other sympathomimetics;
3. The increase in renal blood flow which it produces helps to maintain glomerular filtration rate, urine production and sodium excretion.

Clinical uses and dosage. Dopamine hydrochloride is recommended for treating a number of circulatory decompensation states including shock resulting from trauma, surgery and myocardial infarction; it is also recommended for the treatment of chronic cardiac decompensation as in congestive failure. The commercially available form of the drug (INTROPIN) is a sterile solution containing 40 mg/ml of dopamine hydrochloride in 5 ml ampoules. The contents of the ampoules are diluted with a suitable intravenous fluid such as Dextrose 5 per cent Injection BP to give a solution containing between 400 and 800 micrograms per ml of dopamine hydrochloride. The doses which have been used in man range between 2 and 50 micrograms/kg/minute. It is too early at present to say' whether this substance represents a true advance in the treatment of hypotensive states since it has not yet been fully evaluated in man.

Dobutamine Hydrochloride

This substance which has recently (1977) been introduced into clinical medicine increases cardiac output by selectively stimulating cardiac β_1-adrenoreceptors. It produces little effect on mean arterial blood pressure and is claimed to increase cardiac force at doses which do not increase cardiac rate. Dobutamine therefore is the first sympathomimetic substance selective for β_1-adrenoreceptors and its actions additionally suggest the possibility that cardiac β-adrenoreceptors mediating inotropic effects may differ from those mediating chronotropic responses.

Clinical uses and dosage. Dobutamine is recommended for the treatment in adults of heart failure associated with myocardial infarction, open heart surgery or cardiac myopathies. It is administered by slow intravenous infusion in usual doses of 2·5 to 10 micrograms/kg/minute. It is available in 5 ml ampoules containing 250 mg of the hydrochloride and intended for dilution before use. The proprietary name is DOBUTREX.

General problems associated with the use of pressor drugs to treat hypotensive states

As mentioned earlier in this chapter the value of pressor drugs in the treatment of hypotension is difficult to assess and is an area of controversy. Undoubtedly, badly used, these drugs have the potential to do further harm to patients suffering from a condition in which inadequate tissue perfusion may be the underlying defect. Raising the level of blood pressure in these patients is of dubious value in the absence of correction of hypovolaemia and/or electrolyte imbalance which may also be present. Some of the substances in use, especially the catecholamines, have marked cardiac stimulant effects which usually results in increased myocardial oxygen consumption and may also induce serious disturbances of cardiac rhythm. Many of the substances commonly used are potent vasoconstrictors and they may cause necrosis of surrounding tissues should they leak back from venous injection sites. Substances used by slow intravenous infusion need virtually constant skilled supervision and frequent checks on blood pressure levels to ensure satisfactory results. Those substances, such as metaraminol and mephentermine, with a more prolonged action because of delayed inactivation are more convenient to use since they may be injected in a depot form either subcutaneously or intramuscularly. However, they allow of less precise control of blood pressure and have a tendency to produce diminishing effects on repeated administration (i.e. *tachyphylaxis*).

SYMPATHOMIMETIC SUBSTANCES USED MAINLY TO PRODUCE BRONCHODILATATION

The clinical usage and disadvantages of isoprenaline in the treatment of asthma and related conditions were discussed earlier in this chapter. Various other sympathomimetic substances with β-adrenoreceptor activity have also been used as bronchodilators and some of these are more selective for respiratory tract than cardiovascular system β-adrenoreceptors. Some of the more recently produced drugs such as isoetharine and salbutamol are virtually without cardiovascular effects in doses which markedly reduce airways resistance.

Ephedrine Hydrochloride

$$\underset{\underset{OH}{|}}{CH}-\underset{\underset{CH_3}{|}}{CH}-NH-CH_3 \cdot H\bar{C}l$$

This substance occurs naturally in various species of the plant ephedra which are indigenous to China. Extracts of these plants have been utilised in Chinese medicine for many centuries but it was not until the 1920's that the drug was introduced into Western medicine. Both carbon atoms on the aliphatic side-chain of ephedrine are asymmetric and it follows that four isomeric forms are possible. In practice it is $(-)$-ephedrine, and to a lesser extent the racemic mixture, which is used clinically. The sympathomimetic effects of ephedrine are due to a mixture of direct and indirect actions and of α and β-adrenoreceptor stimulation. It is only slowly metabolised in the body which results in it being effective orally, having a prolonged duration and allows it to penetrate into the brain where it causes stimulant effects resembling, but weaker than, those of amphetamine.

Ephedrine raises arterial blood pressure by virtue of its α-effect in causing vasoconstriction and its β-effect in stimulating the heart. It has a small and variable effect on the heart rate and causes coronary vasodilatation. It is less potent than either adrenaline or isoprenaline in causing bronchodilatation but its action is more prolonged than either and it has the added advantage of being fully active by the oral route.

Clinical uses and dosage. Ephedrine has been used for all the clinical conditions in which sympathomimetic substances are effective but its most important action is for the prophylactic treatment of bronchospasm. Ephedrine Hydrochloride BP is the

(−)-isomer and it is used orally in adult doses of 15 to 60 mg repeated 3 to 4 times daily for treating milder forms of asthma. It is much less effective in treating bronchospasm once it has occurred and more rapidly acting substances are generally used in emergency states.

Ephedrine has been used intramuscularly to raise arterial blood pressure in hypotensive states but it is subject to tachyphylaxis and is probably inferior to other available pressor agents. It is sometimes used orally in doses of 15 to 30 mg up to three times daily to treat heart block associated with fainting (Stokes-Adams attacks).

Solutions containing 2 to 5 per cent ephedrine hydrochloride are used in ophthalmology as a mydriatic and preparations and drops containing 0·5 to 2 per cent are used topically to relieve nasal congestion in hay fever and related allergic conditions.

Ephedrine Hydrochloride Tablets BP, BNF each contain 30 mg of active constituent. Ephedrine Elixir BPC, BNF contains 15 mg of the hydrochloride in each 5 ml and is a preparation particularly suited for use in children. Ephedrine Nasal Drops BPC, BNF contain 0·5 per cent of the hydrochloride. Ephedrine is a constituent of a number of proprietary preparations which often contain in addition barbiturates and/or antihistamines and which are used orally for the treatment of chronic bronchitis and allergic conditions such as hay fever.

β-adrenoreceptor stimulants selective for the respiratory tract

Isoprenaline is equally effective in stimulating bronchial and cardiac β-adrenoreceptors whilst ephedrine, although less active at both sites, has a slight selectivity for effects on the respiratory system. This differing activity on β-adrenoreceptors at different sites is shown even more clearly by methoxyphenamine, a substance, structurally related to ephedrine, first used in man in 1948. In 1967 Lands, Arnold, McAuliff, Luduena and Brown analysed the sensitivity of β-adrenoreceptors in various tissues to stimulation by β-agonists and they concluded that β-adrenoreceptors could be further subdivided into two distinct groups. They called the receptors in the heart and small intestine β_1 and those in the bronchi, vascular beds and uterus β_2. This sub-classification has been of considerable value in the development of both selective β_2-adrenoreceptor agonists such as salbutamol and also of selective β_1-adrenoreceptor antagonists (see Chapter 12). The structural formulae and names of the

Table 9.4 Structural formulae of sympathomimetic drugs with β_2-adrenoreceptor stimulant activity which are used as bronchodilators.

Structural formula	Name	Proprietary name(s)
$CH_2-CH-NH-CH_3$, CH_3, OCH_3	methoxyphenamine	ORTHOXINE
HO, HO, $CH-CH_2-NH-CH$, OH, CH_3, CH_3	orciprenaline	ALUPENT
HO, HO, $CH-CH-NH\cdot CH$, OH C_2H_5, CH_3, CH_3	isoetharine	NUMOTAC BRONCHILATOR (in combination with other drugs)
$HOCH_2$, HO, $CH-CH_2-NH-C-CH_3$, OH, CH_3, CH_3	salbutamol	VENTOLIN
HO, HO, $CH-CH_2-NH-C-CH_3$, OH, CH_3, CH_3	terbutaline	BRICANYL, FILAIR
HO, HO, CH, OH N H	rimiterol	PULMADIL

selective β_2-adrenoreceptor stimulants at present in clinical use in the United Kingdom are shown in Table 9.4.

Methoxyphenamine Hydrochloride

This substance is chemically related to ephedrine but is a more potent bronchodilator and has weaker effects on the cardio-vascular and central nervous systems. It is virtually devoid of α-adrenoreceptor stimulant activity.

Clinical uses and dosage. The indications for methoxyphen-amine are similar to those for ephedrine. It is used in the treatment of chronic bronchial asthma and is useful in patients intolerant to ephedrine. It is also effective in the treatment of allergic rhinitis and acute urticaria. The usual adult oral dose is

50 to 100 mg repeated 3 or 4 hourly. It is available commercially as tablets containing 100 mg (ORTHOXINE).

Orciprenaline Sulphate BP

This substance differs chemically from isoprenaline only in the position of one of the hydroxy groups on the benzene ring. It differs pharmacologically from isoprenaline in being more selective for the β_2-adrenoreceptors of the respiratory tract, in having a more prolonged duration of action and in being more completely absorbed by mouth.

Clinical uses and dosage. The usual adult oral dose of orciprenaline is 80 mg per day usually in divided doses. For more rapid effects it may be administered by inhalation or by subcutaneous or intramuscular injection. Official preparations of orciprenaline are Orciprenaline Tablets BP, BNF which each contain 20 mg of the sulphate, Orciprenaline Elixir, BPC, BNF which contains 10 mg in 5 ml, Orciprenaline Injection BP which contains 0·5 mg per ml and Orciprenaline Aerosol Inhalation BPC, BNF which delivers metered doses of 750 micrograms (maximum dose, 12 inhalations in 24 hours). The proprietary name for orciprenaline sulphate is ALUPENT.

β_2-adrenoreceptor stimulants inhibit uterine muscle contraction and they have been used by slow intravenous infusion to inhibit premature labour. The intravenous dose of orciprenaline sulphate used in obstetrics for this purpose is usually in the range of 15 to 25 micrograms per minute.

Isoetharine Hydrochloride

This compound is the α-ethyl derivative of isoprenaline and was one of the compounds shown by Lands and his colleagues to be selective for β_2-adrenoreceptors. It is effective by mouth but its action is short due to rapid inactivation in the body mainly by catechol-O-methyltransferase.

Clinical uses and dosage. For oral administration isoetharine is administered in 10 mg delayed release tablets (NUMOTAC) which give an effective duration of action of 4 to 6 hours. The daily dose in this form is 30 to 40 mg. Isoetharine is also a constituent of an aerosol preparation (BRONCHILATOR) which delivers a metered dose of 350 micrograms of isoetharine hydrochloride.

Salbutamol Sulphate BP

This compound is probably the most widely used β_2-adrenoreceptor stimulant available. It is effective by all routes of administration, has a much longer duration of action than isoprenaline and is virtually devoid of cardiovascular effects in usual human doses. It is not metabolized by catechol-O-methyl-transferase.

Clinical uses and dosage. The oral dose in the treatment of bronchial asthma is 2 to 4 mg three times daily. For administration by inhalation from aerosol containers the dose is 100 to 200 micrograms repeated 4 hourly with a maximum of 8 inhalations in 24 hours. Salbutamol has been used by slow intravenous infusion (10 to 45 micrograms min) to inhibit uterine contractions in premature labour.

Salbutamol Tablets BP, BNF contain either 2 or 4 mg of the sulphate and Salbutamol Aerosol Inhalation BPC, BNF contains 200 metered doses each of 100 micrograms. It is available in a variety of forms including an injection for intravenous use under the proprietary name of VENTOLIN.

Terbutaline Sulphate
This substance is closely related chemically to orciprenaline but is reputedly slightly more β_2-selective.

Clinical use and dosage. The oral dose of terbutaline is 2·5 to 5 mg two or three times daily. It may also be administered by subcutaneous injection (250 to 500 micrograms) or by inhalation (200 or 250 micrograms metered doses). It is available commercially under the proprietary names of BRICANYL and FILAIR.

Rimiterol Hydrobromide
This is a very short acting β_2-adrenoreceptor stimulant, not active by mouth, but which produces a potent bronchodilator effect of rapid onset and short duration when administered by inhalation.

Clinical use and dosage. It is administered by inhalation from an aerosol preparation delivering 200 micrograms metered doses (PULMADIL).

Ritodrine Hydrochloride

$$HO-\langle\bigcirc\rangle-\underset{\underset{OH}{|}}{CH}-\underset{\underset{CH_3}{|}}{CH}-NH-CH_2-CH_2-\langle\bigcirc\rangle-OH\cdot HCl$$

Ritodrine is a recently introduced selective β_2-adrenoreceptor stimulant which is recommended solely for its action in relaxing uterine smooth muscle and thereby of delaying parturition.

Clinical use and dosage. Ritodrine is used to treat premature labour in which condition it is used initially by slow intravenous infusion in a commencing dose of 50 micrograms/minute which may be gradually increased up to a maximum of 350 micrograms/minute. Once labour has been arrested then a more prolonged action may be achieved by either the intramuscular (10 mg three hourly) or oral (10 mg every two to six hours) route. It is commercially available under the name of YUTOPAR as an injection containing 10 mg/ml of the hydrochloride or as tablets of 10 mg strength.

General precautions in the use of β_2-adrenoreceptor stimulants

Initial clinical studies using β_2-selective substances indicated that they are effective in the treatment of reversible airways obstruction such as occurs in bronchial asthma and chronic bronchitis and that they produce less cardiovascular side-effects such as changes in blood pressure, tachycardia and palpitations than older remedies such as adrenaline and isoprenaline. Moreover, sudden deaths amongst asthmatics have declined with the reduction in the usage of aerosol preparations containing isoprenaline. However, it should be remembered that all of the β_2-selective substances in use can, in sufficient dosage, produce cardiovascular effects and their indiscriminate use, particularly in aerosol formulations, would be unwise until they have been in clinical use for a much longer period. As with all sympathomimetics particular caution should be exercised when these substances are used in patients suffering from cardiovascular disorders or from thyrotoxicosis and also in patients receiving other drugs, such as monoamine oxidase inhibitors, which may produce adverse drug interactions with sympathomimetics.

The β_2-selective substances commonly cause a tremor of skeletal muscles in patients receiving them as bronchodilators. This effect is due to stimulation of β_2-adrenoreceptors in skeletal muscles which increases the rate of skeletal muscle relaxation and thus amplifies the normal physiological tremor. The effect is most marked with oral preparations and is seldom a problem with drugs administered by inhalation.

SYMPATHOMIMETICS USED MAINLY AS NASAL DECONGESTANTS

A number of sympathomimetic substances have been used both systemically and by topical application to induce vasoconstriction* of inflamed mucous membranes and thus produce symptomatic relief of nasal congestion in allergic conditions and also in the treatment of the common cold. In general these substances are α-adrenoreceptor stimulants and the structures of some of those still in clinical use are shown in Table 9.5.

Table 9.5 Structural formulae of sympathomimetics with α-adrenoreceptor stimulant activity and used mainly to produce nasal decongestion.

Structural formula	Name	Proprietary name(s)
CH—CH—NH$_2$ / OH CH$_3$	phenylpropanolamine	TRIOMINIC ESKORNADE (both in combination with other drugs)
HO— CH$_2$—CH—NH$_2$ / CH$_3$	hydroxyamphetamine	VASOCORT (in combination with other drugs)
—CH$_2$— (naphazoline ring)	naphazoline	PRIVINE
H$_3$C, H$_3$C—C, H$_3$C — CH$_3$ — CH$_2$ — CH$_3$	xylometazoline	OTRIVINE

Phenylpropanolamine Hydrochloride BPC

This substance is a potent α-adrenoreceptor stimulant and is used both orally and by topical application. In the treatment of allergic rhinitis it is used in oral doses up to 50 mg and it is a constituent of several proprietary preparations which also contain analgesics and/or antihistamines and which are used to treat similar conditions. When used orally it may sometimes increase arterial blood pressure and there have been reports of dangerous pressor responses induced by it in patients concurrently receiving monoamine oxidase inhibitors. It has been used by parenteral routes to treat hypotension but there are more suitable drugs available. It may produce some stimulant effects on the brain resembling those of amphetamine and it may be this property which is at least partly responsible for the subjective improvement of patients taking the drug to treat the common cold.

It is applied topically to the nasal mucosa in solutions containing 1·5 per cent of the hydrochloride in the treatment of allergic rhinitis.

Hydroxyamphetamine Hydrobromide

This substance resembles phenylpropanolamine both in chemical structure and pharmacological effects. It was formerly used to raise blood pressure but is now almost entirely used by local application as a nasal decongestant.

Naphazoline nitrate and Xylometazoline hydrochloride

These substances have very similar actions and both are α-adrenoreceptor stimulants derived from imidazoline. Other derivatives of imidazoline such as tolazoline (Chapter 11) are α-adrenoreceptor blocking drugs whilst clonidine (Chapter 13) is another derivative which although a potent α-adrenoreceptor stimulant reduces arterial pressure às a result of an action on the hindbrain.

Naphazoline and xylometazoline are each used as 0·1 per cent solutions in the form of nasal sprays to treat nasal congestion.

Precautions with substances used as nasal decongestants

Some sympathomimetic substances used orally as nasal decongestants may produce dangerous rises in blood pressure. Increases in blood pressure and drowsiness have also been reported as side-effects of topical application of the imidazoline derivatives. It has also been reported that the repeated application of vasoconstrictor substances to produce nasal decongestion can lead to severe 'rebound congestion' such that on discontinuance of treatment the congestion may be as bad as, or even worse than, before treatment. For this reason the long-term use of these preparations should be discouraged.

Isoxuprine Hydrochloride

$$HO-\langle \bigcirc \rangle-\underset{\underset{OH}{|}}{CH}-\underset{\underset{CH_3}{|}}{CH}-NH-\underset{\underset{CH_3}{|}}{CH}-CH_2-O-\langle \bigcirc \rangle \cdot H\bar{C}l$$

This compound is of interest because it is a β-adrenoreceptor stimulant which is used to produce dilatation of peripheral blood vessels in conditions associated with excessive vasoconstriction and poor peripheral blood flow such as Raynaud's disease. The drug is thought to act mainly on β-adrenoreceptors in small arteries and arterioles supplying skeletal muscle and to produce little dilator effect on vessels in the splanchnic area. It would appear that isoxuprine has some selectivity for β_2-adrenoreceptors since it produces little effect on either cardiac rate or systemic arterial blood pressure; it may also be a weak α-adrenoreceptor antagonist which would tend to increase its vasodilator action.

Clinical uses and dosage. Isoxuprine is effective orally and up to 20 mg repeated 3 or 4 times daily has been used in the treatment of peripheral occlusive vascular disorders such as Raynaud's disease, thrombophlebitis, ischaemic ulcers and Buerger's disease. It is also said to increase cerebral blood flow in patients suffering from cerebral arteriosclerosis. Its duration of action is about 2 hours but is increased to 6-8 hours by delayed release preparations.

It is available commercially as tablets each containing 20 mg of the hydrochloride (DUVADILAN, VASOTRAN), as delayed release tablets containing 40 mg (DUVADILAN RETARD, DEFENCIN) and also in an injectable form for intramuscular use containing 10 mg in 2 ml.

Amphetamines and derivatives

As mentioned earlier in this chapter the central actions of amphetamine and its derivatives are beyond the scope of this monograph. However, these substances may have important pharmacological effects outside of the central nervous system particularly when used in high doses by persons using them for their mood-elevating effects. Thus fatalities have occurred from cerebrovascular haemorrhages resulting from the marked and sustained increases in blood pressure caused by high doses of these substances. Amphetamine and some of its derivatives are used clinically to treat obesity and they may have an important peripheral effect in antagonising the pharmacological action of noradrenergic neurone blocking drugs which are used to treat hypertension. This interaction is described more fully in the next chapter.

INTERACTION OF SYMPATHOMIMETIC SUBSTANCES WITH MONOAMINE OXIDASE INHIBITING DRUGS

Monoamine oxidase inhibiting drugs are used mainly in the treatment of severe mental depression; however, like amphetamine and its derivatives, they also have important peripheral actions. As a result of inhibiting intraneuronal monoamine oxidase the level of noradrenaline present in many peripheral noradrenergic neurones is elevated. In addition some sympathomimetic substances which are normally degraded by monoamine oxidase will persist in the body for much longer periods following its inhibition. This drug interaction is of particular consequence in the case of sympathomimetics which are both

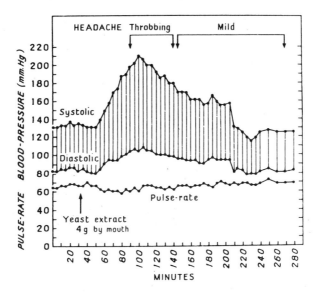

Fig. 9.5 Effect of eating 4 g of a yeast extract (MARMITE) on the blood pressure and pulse rate of a woman concurrently receiving the monoamine oxidase inhibiting drug tranylcypromine (PARNATE) for the treatment of depression. (From Blackwell, Marley & Mabbitt, 1965).

metabolised by monoamine oxidase and which produce their pharmacological effects indirectly by releasing neuronal noradrenaline. Two such substances are phenylethylamine and tyramine which are present in many foodstuffs and which normally do not produce pharmacological effects when taken in the diet. However, following inhibition of monoamine oxidase these substances may be absorbed into the bloodstream in sufficient concentration to cause dangerous increases in blood pressure often associated with palpitations and a severe headache. This interaction is illustrated in Fig. 9.5; it is dangerous because it may precipitate a fatal cerebral haemorrhage or even acute cardiac failure. Foodstuffs containing a high proportion of tyramine are cheese, especially if well matured, pickled herrings, yeast extracts such as MARMITE and BOVRIL and some wines and beers. Broad beans have also been reported to produce a similar syndrome after inhibition of monoamine oxidase and in this case the amino-acid L-DOPA has been implicated.

SUMMARY

Sympathomimetic substances produce effects in the body which broadly resemble the effects produced by stimulation of the sympathetic nervous system. These effects may be induced by stimulation of α and/or β-adrenoreceptors by either a direct action on the receptors or indirectly via release of neuronal noradrenaline stores. In practice α and β-adrenoreceptor stimulant activity and direct and indirect activity form continuous spectra such that no substance is wholly selective for one site or type of action.

The majority of sympathomimetics in clinical use are derived from phenylethylamine and predictable changes in activity occur in many of these compounds with change in chemical structure. Addition of hydroxyl groups in the 3- and 4-positions on the benzene ring and on the β-carbon atom of the aliphatic side-chain increase the overall sympathomimetic effects of phenylethylamine and change its action qualitatively from mainly indirect to mainly direct. The addition of a hydroxyl group to the 3-position on the benzene ring is more important that hydroxylation of the 4-position in terms of both increased overall sympathomimetic activity and of direct rather than indirect activity. Alkyl substituents on the amine group of phenylethylamine and its derivatives increases β-adreno-receptor stimulant activity at the expense of α-activity. Addition of a methyl group to the α-carbon atom of the aliphatic side-chain of phenylethylamine derivatives render them immune to oxidative deamination by monoamine oxidase.

Sympathomimetic substances are used clinically mainly for their actions on the cardiovascular and respiratory systems. Substances with mainly α-adrenoreceptor stimulant activity are used to raise arterial blood pressure in hypotensive states occurring for example as a sequel to surgical shock or myocardial infarction. These substances raise blood pressure mainly by producing vasoconstriction and most have little effect on cardiac output unless this is severely reduced. The effectiveness of these substances in aiding recovery from hypotensive states is difficult to assess and a subject of controversy. Modern therapy of hypotension places great emphasis on correcting hypovolaemia and/or electrolyte balance and less on the actual level of arterial blood pressure. Sympathomimetic drugs used to raise blood pressure include noradrenaline, metaraminol, methoxamine and phenylephrine.

Sympathomimetic substances with predominantly β-adreno-receptor stimulant activity are used to relax the smooth muscle of the respiratory tract in conditions such as asthma characterised by bronchoconstriction. However, some β-adrenoreceptor stimulants such as isoprenaline may cause marked effects on the cardiovascular system including cardiac stimulation and peripheral vasodilatation in doses needed to produce bronchodilatation. Chemical modifications of the isoprenaline structure have led to the introduction of substances which produce bronchodilatation at doses producing minimal effects on the cardiovascular system. These substances have led to a reclassification of β-adrenoreceptors into two sub-groups: those in the heart and intestine have been designated β_1 and those in the respiratory tract, vasculature and uterus β_2. β_2-adrenoreceptor stimulants which are used clinically to produce bronchodilatation include orciprenaline, salbutamol and isoetharine.

Sympathomimetic substances have a number of other clinical uses such as producing local vasoconstriction to relieve nasal congestion in allergic and related conditions, to reduce local haemorrhage, to produce mydriasis without cyclopegia and to relax the uterus in cases of premature labour. Sympathomimetics related to amphetamine have important stimulant effects on the brain and also produce anorexia; these substances are used in the treatment of obesity. Sympathomimetic substances with marked central actions also have peripheral actions and may interact peripherally with other drugs. Many sympathomimetics, including some naturally occurring amines present in foodstuffs, produce enhanced effects in patients receiving mono-amine oxidase inhibiting drugs; this interaction may have important clinical consequences.

REFERENCES

Ahlquist, R. P. (1948) A study of adrenotropic receptors. *Amer. J. Physiol.*, **153**, 586–600.
Allwood, M. J., Cobbold, A. F. & Ginsburg, J. (1963) Peripheral vascular effects of noradrenaline, isopropylnoradrenaline and dopamine. *Br. med. Bull.*, **19**, 132–136.

Barger, G. & Dale, H. H. (1910) Chemical structure and sympathomimetic action of amines. *J. Physiol.*, **41**, 19–59.

Belleau, B. (1963) An analysis of drug receptor interactions. In *Modern Concepts in the Relationship between Structure and Pharmacological Activity, Proceedings of the First International Pharmacological Meeting, 1961.* Vol. 7, 75–99, London: Pergamon Press.

Bertler, A., Carlsson, A. & Rosengren, E. (1956) Release by reserpine of catecholamines from rabbits' hearts. *Naturwissenschaften*, **43**, 521.

Blackwell, B., Marley, E. & Mabbit, L. A. (1965) Effects of yeast extract after monoamine oxidase inhibition. *Lancet*, **1**, 940–943.

Burn, J. H. & Rand, M. J. (1958) The action of sympathomimetic amines in animals treated with reserpine. *J. Physiol.*, **144**, 314–346.

Burn, J. H. & Tainter, M. L. (1931) An analysis of the effect of cocaine on the actions of adrenaline and tyramine. *J. Physiol.*, **71**, 169–193.

Innes, I. R. & Nickerson, M. (1975) Norepinephrine, epinephrine and the sympathomimetic amines. In *The Pharmacological Basis of Therapeutics*, 5th edn., pp. 477–513, ed. Goodman, L. S. & Gilman, A. New York: Macmillan Publishing Co.

Kunos, G. & Nickerson, M. (1976) Temperature-induced inter-conversion of α- and β-adrenoreceptors in the frog heart. *J. Physiol.*, **256**, 23–40.

Lands, A. M., Arnold, A., McAuliff, J. P., Luduena, F. P. & Brown, T. G., Jr. (1967) Differentiation of receptor systems activated by sympathomimetic amines. *Nature, Lond.*, **214**, 597–598.

Tainter, M. L. & Chang, D. K. (1927) The antagonism of the pressor action of tyramine by cocaine. *J. Pharmac. exp. Ther.*, **39**, 193–207.

GENERAL READING

Aviado, D. M. (1970) *Sympathomimetic Drugs.* Springfield: Charles C. Thomas.

Foster, R. W. (1966) The pharmacology of pressor drugs. *Br. J. Anaesth.*, **38**, 690–704.

Lands, A. M. & Brown, T. G. (1967) Sympathomimetic (adrenergic) stimulants. In *Drugs Affecting the Peripheral Nervous System* Vol. 1, pp. 399–472, ed. Burger, A. London: Edward Arnold Ltd.

Marley, E. & Blackwell, B. (1970) Interactions of monoamine oxidase inhibitors amines and foodstuffs. *Adv. Pharmac. Chemother.*, **8**, 185–239.

Martindale, (1977). *The Extra Pharmacopoeia* 27th edn., London: The Pharmaceutical Press.

Rand, M. J. & Trinker, F. R. (1966) Pharmacological agents affecting the release and activity of catecholamines. *Br. J. Anaesth.*, **38**, 666–689.

Smith, N. T. & Corbascio, A. N. (1970) The use and misuse of pressor agents. *Anaesthesiology*, **33**, 58–101.

Zaimis, E. (1968) Vasopressor drugs and catecholamines. *Anaesthesiology*, **29**, 732–762.

10

Noradrenergic neurone blocking drugs

The ganglion blocking drugs which block transmission in sympathetic nerves by competition with acetylcholine for nicotinic receptors in autonomic ganglia were described in Chapter 7. These drugs were formerly much used to lower arterial blood pressure in patients suffering from hypertension. However, in clinical use ganglion blockers produce a formidable number of unwanted actions and accordingly attempts were made to produce drugs which would block transmission only in sympathetic ganglia. These attempts failed but a new class of drug was discovered whose primary action is to prevent the release of noradrenaline from sympathetic nerves without blocking post synaptic adrenoreceptors in effector tissues. These drugs have major clinical advantages over ganglion blockers in not impairing transmission in either the parasympathetic system or in sympathetic cholinergic nerves and in thus producing a narrower spectrum of unwanted actions. Drugs of this type are often referred to as adrenergic neurone blockers but in this monograph the more accurate term noradrenergic neurone blocker will be used.

Xylocholine (TM10)

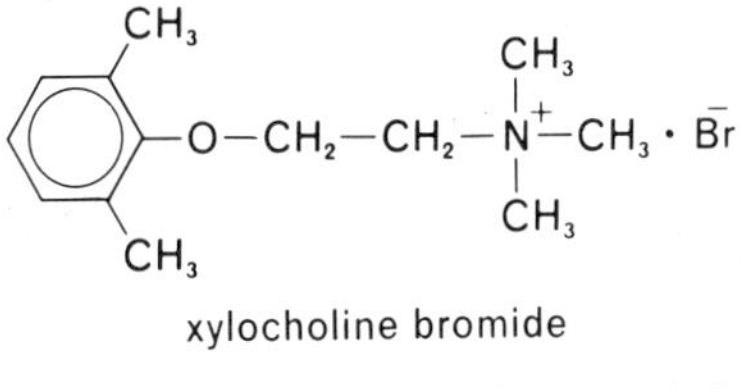

xylocholine bromide

This compound was the forerunner of the noradrenergic neurone blocking agents and was first described by Hey & Willey (1954) who gave it the identification number of TM10 by which it is often known to pharmacologists. Chemically, TM10 is the 2:6-xylyl ether of choline and thus is structurally related to acetylcholine. It stimulates and may also block both muscarinic and nicotinic acetylcholine receptors and has a number of other pharmacological properties including a potent local anaesthetic action and a weak inhibitory effect on monoamine oxidase. However, the most interesting property of the compound is its ability to produce a slowly developing but persistent blockade of the responses to sympathetic nerve stimulation. Exley (1957)

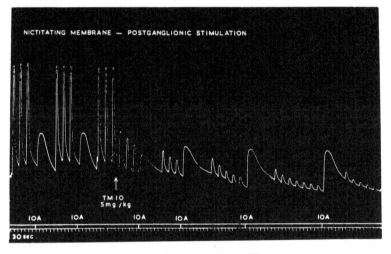

Fig. 10.1 Noradrenergic neurone blocking action of TM10 on the nictitating membrane of an anaesthetised cat.
The contractions of the membrane in response to intermittent electrical stimulation of its postganglionic sympathetic nerve trunk were almost abolished by an intravenous injection of TM10 (5 mg/Kg). However, the contractions of the membrane in response to 10 microgram doses of adrenaline were slightly reduced at first but later were at least as large as the responses before TM10. (From Exley, 1957).

demonstrated that the blockade of the responses to sympathetic stimulation produced by TM10 on the cat's nictitating membrane was not due to an adrenoreceptor blocking action since the contractions of the membrane to intravenously administered adrenaline were only transiently reduced and were in fact increased above control level at the time of maximum impairment of the nervously-mediated responses (see Fig. 10.1). Exley also showed that TM10 markedly reduced the release of noradrenaline in response to electrical stimulation of the splenic (sympathetic) nerves but did not reduce the release of catecholamines from the adrenal medullae in response to splanchnic nerve stimulation.

TM10 was tested in man and was found to lower the blood pressure of hypertensive patients but its wide spectrum of pharmacological actions precluded its general use to treat this condition.

Bretylium

bretylium tosylate

The lead provided by TM10 led to the synthesis of a number of compounds with similar actions on sympathetic nerves and the first of these to be used as an antihypertensive agent in man was bretylium. The pharmacological properties of bretylium were first described by Boura & Green (1959) who showed that it selectively blocked the responses to sympathetic nerve stimulation in a variety of smooth muscle tissues. Bretylium produced no effect on responses elicited by stimulation of cholinergic sympathetic nerves such as those innervating the sweat glands of the skin nor did it reduce the release of catecholamines from the adrenal medullae in response to splanchnic nerve stimulation. Bretylium, unlike TM10, has fewer other pharmacological actions on peripheral tissues; after intravenous injection it causes an initial sympathomimetic effect which is apparently due to acute displacement of noradrenaline from sympathetic nerves and in high doses it reduces the effects of acetylcholine at both muscarinic and nicotinic sites. Like TM10, bretylium has local anaesthetic activity and its pharmacological effects are confined to the periphery and it produces no obvious effects on the central nervous system.

Therapeutic use of bretylium. The results of the initial clinical trials using bretylium to treat human hypertension were encouraging. It was found to produce a mainly orthostatic lowering of blood pressure similar to that occurring with ganglion blocking drugs but without the effects such as dry mouth and constipation attributable to parasympathetic blockade. In general, the side-effects produced by bretylium when used to treat hypertension were those predictable from a non-selective blockade of sympathetic nerves and included nasal stuffiness, diarrhoea, postural hypotension and failure of ejaculation in the male. The most disturbing effects arose from the abolition of circulatory reflexes which led to severe postural hypotension on standing from a lying position and also hypotension occurring on muscular exercise. However, the problem which led to the abandonment of bretylium as an antihypertensive drug was the tendency for many patients to become more or less rapidly tolerant to its effects requiring frequent and sometimes impractical increases in dosage. It is not entirely clear why this tolerance occurs although it seems to be related to the increase in the responsiveness to circulating noradrenaline which bretylium induces. It has also been shown that bretylium is more effective in preventing release of noradrenaline from sympathetic nerves in response to high frequencies of nerve stimulation; low frequency stimulation being relatively much less effected. Since physiological rates of impulse traffic in sympathetic nerves are believed to be low it follows that these are least affected by bretylium and, with the supersensitivity to noradrenaline which develops with chronic bretylium treatment, a situation may occur in which a reduced amount of transmitter released from sympathetic nerves may produce effects equivalent to those produced by much higher amounts before treatment. Another disadvantage of bretylium is that it is irregularly and incompletely absorbed from the intestine when given by mouth and thus its effects on blood pressure may be unpredictable even in patients in whom tolerance is not a problem.

Bretylium is no longer used as an antihypertensive drug but it has recently been marketed in an injectable form for the treatment of ventricular arrhythmias. For this use it is available as 2 ml ampoules each containing 50 mg per ml of bretylium tosylate (BRETYLATE). It is administered by the intramuscular route in an initial dose of 5 mg/kg body weight which may be repeated at intervals of 6 to 8 hours. It is not yet clear what the mechanism of the antiarrhythymic effect of bretylium is although it is likely that its local anaesthetic action is involved.

Guanethidine

guanethidine sulphate

The actions of this substance were first described by Maxwell, Mull & Plummer (1959) shortly after, but apparently independent of, the introduction of bretylium. Guanethidine bears only a superficial chemical resemblance to either TM10 or bretylium although like both it is a strongly basic substance and at physiological pH the nitrogen atom bears a strong positive charge. The effect of guanethidine on noradrenergic nerve function was discovered largely as a result of the prolonged abolition of cardiovascular reflexes which it produced in anaesthetised dogs. It was found that in dogs some degree of sympathetic nerve impairment persisted for 5 to 20 days after a single intravenous dose of guanethidine and that it reduced the arterial blood pressure of both normotensive and hypertensive dogs. In many respects the pharmacology of guanethidine closely resembles that of bretylium. Thus it selectively prevents the release of noradrenaline from noradrenergic nerves without reducing the effects of exogenously administered noradrenaline on effector tissues. It does not affect the functioning of sympathetic cholinergic nerves or the release of catecholamines from the adrenal medullae in response to splanchnic nerve stimulation. Also, like bretylium, it is a potent local anaesthetic, produces initial sympathomimetic effects after intravenous injection, increases the responses to circulating or injected noradrenaline and in high doses has weak anti-acetylcholine activity. The major differences of practical importance between the actions of bretylium and guanethidine are that guanethidine is much more potent, has a much longer duration of action and tolerance to its effects on repeated dosage rarely occurs. In some animal experiments in which high doses of guanethidine were used it was shown to have a more marked action that either TM10 or bretylium in reducing peripheral neuronal stores of noradrenaline. However, it is unlikely that this difference is fundamental to its mode of action in man. Other animal studies have shown that prolonged treatment with guanethidine can produce permanent damage to noradrenergic neurones such that a functional partial sympathectomy may be produced. The relevance of this observation to the clinical use of the drug is unclear.

Therapeutic use of guanethidine. The major clinical use for guanethidine is in the treatment of severe hypertension. It was formerly used in all grades of hypertension but with the introduction of drugs with fewer side-effects such as the β-adrenoreceptor blockers (Chapter 12) and α-methyldopa (Chapter 13), its use is now restricted to the treatment of severe hypertension particularly in patients where milder drugs have been found to be ineffective. The mechanism of its antihypertensive effect is partly due to a fall in peripheral resistance resulting from abolition of vasoconstrictor sympathetic tone and partly to a fall in cardiac output resulting from reduced venous return due to venodilatation. The drug is usually administered by mouth but it is only absorbed to an extent of 10-20 per cent by this route. However, its absorption is more regular than that of bretylium and consequently its effects on blood pressure are more predictable. The effects of guanethidine in man have been shown to be as persistent as they are in animals, signs of sympathetic impairment remaining for up to 3 weeks after discontinuing the drug. This prolonged action of guanethidine makes fine adjustment of dose in individual patients difficult but means that in many patients once a day treatment is adequate to control blood pressure. The side-effects of guanethidine are similar to those of bretylium with postural and exertional hypotension the most troublesome together with a much increased tendency over bretylium to cause diarrhoea. As with bretylium the degree of hypotension produced by guanethidine is dependent on the amount of traffic in peripheral sympathetic nerves which is much greater in the standing than in the lying position. However, because of the prolonged action of guanethidine marked postural hypotension can be particularly troublesome to the patient when some degree of venous pooling has occurred as for example after a night's rest in bed. For this reason in patients receiving guanethidine feelings of dizziness and nausea sometimes accompanied by fainting are particularly common on rising and these effects are made worse by warm weather. It has also been shown that very marked fluctuations in blood pressure .may occur during the course of a day, spells of very low blood pressure being associated with exertion. Many patients receiving guanethidine complain of a general feeling of lassitude which may be partly due to periods of very low blood pressure although a blocking effect on the skeletal neuromuscular junction and a reduction in the release of free fatty acids from adipose tissue have also been implicated.

When used to treat hypertension guanethidine and the other drugs of this type have been shown to produce oedema in some patients due to retention of sodium and water. This effect may be abolished by the concurrent administration of a thiazide diuretic such as chlorothiazide. The thiazides also have a useful effect in potentiating the antihypertensive effects of guanethidine and thus allowing of a reduction in dosage with a consequent reduction in the incidence of side-effects.

Guanethidine when applied locally to the eye has been found to be useful in the treatment of glaucoma. This effect is believed to be due to a reduction in the production of aqueous humour resulting from blockade of sympathetic nerves. The effect of guanethidine in producing this effect is at first puzzling since, as stated in the previous chapter, adrenaline is used to decrease production of aqueous humour and therefore it would be expected that guanethidine would produce the opposite effect. However, Bron (1969) has suggested that increase in flow of aqueous humour is mediated by α-adrenoreceptors and inhibition by β-adrenoreceptors. The observations can therefore be reconciled by postulating that guanethidine decreases flow by inhibiting the effects of sympathetic neurones stimulating α-adrenoreceptors whilst the useful effect of adrenaline is due to β-adrenoreceptor stimulation.

Dosage and preparations of guanethidine. In the treatment of severe hypertension guanethidine is given by mouth in a usual starting dose of 10 to 20 mg per day. The full effects of treatment may take up to a week to develop and the dose is usually adjusted by weekly increments of 10 mg. The usual maintenance dose is 50 to 75 mg per day but up to 400 mg have been used.

The official (BP, BNF) tablets each contain 10 mg of guanethidine sulphate BP unless another strength is specified. The proprietary form of the drug (ISMELIN) is available in tablets of 10 or 25 mg strength and an injectable form containing 10 mg in 1 ml ampoules. Guanethidine is occasionally used by intramuscular injection in doses of 10 to 20 mg in hypertensive crises such as may occur in toxaemia of pregnancy. Guanethidine (10 mg) is also available combined with cyclopenthiazide (150 micrograms and potassium chloride (400 mg) in a proprietary tablet preparation (ISMELIN-NAVIDREX K).

Guanethidine in the form of eye-drops is used to treat glaucoma and also to relax the upper eyelids when these are retracted in patients suffering from thyrotoxicosis. The usual strength of eye-drops (BNF) is 5 per cent which is also the strength of the proprietary preparation (ISMELIN).

Bethanidine

bethanidine sulphate

Bethanidine is chemically related to both bretylium and guanethidine and pharmacologically it also falls between the other two agents. Thus, like bretylium, it is short-acting and less likely to cause profound hypotension in the morning and it causes diarrhoea much less often or severely than guanethidine. It resembles guanethidine in being potent and in having little tendency to induce tolerance on repeated dosage. It is unlike either bretylium or guanethidine in being well absorbed from the intestine after oral administration. It is mostly excreted in the urine within 24 hours of administration and so is unlikely to produce cumulative effects. After oral administration bethanidine starts to lower blood pressure within 1 to 2 hours and produces its peak effects within 4 to 5 hours; its effects have usually completely subsided within 12 hours of administration. The pharmacological effects of bethanidine are essentially similar to those of the other noradrenergic neurone blocking agents and differences in its effects in man from other agents are quantitative rather than qualitative.

Clinical use and dosage. Bethanidine, like the other drugs in this class, tends to be reserved for patients with severe hypertension. The usual starting dose is 10 to 20 mg per day in divided doses and this may be adjusted by increments of 5 to 10 mg per day until the desired effect on blood pressure is achieved. The usual maintenance dose is 20 to 200 mg per day. Some tolerance to bethanidine is quite common but this is not rapidly progressive as it is with bretylium and can usually be easily dealt with by adjustment of the dose. Bethanidine is administered orally in tablets (BP, BNF) containing 10 or 50 mg in each. It is also available in tablets of the same strength under the proprietary name of ESBATAL.

Bethanidine is probably the easiest drug of this class to use. Its short duration of action and good oral absorption make it relatively easy for the physician to rapidly arrive at a suitable dose level. The reduced tendency of the drug to cause diarrhoea and early morning postural hypotension are positive advantages from the patient's viewpoint.

Debrisoquine

debrisoquine sulphate

This compound closely resembles bethanidine both chemically and in the pharmacological effects which it produces. Like bethanidine it is well absorbed by mouth and mostly excreted in the urine within 24 hours. Its onset of action is perhaps slightly more rapid than bethanidine reaching a peak effect in 2 to 3 hours.

Clinical uses and dosage. The indications for debrisoquine are the same as for bethanidine; the oral starting dose is 20 mg per day in divided doses and maintenance doses range between 20 and 150 mg per day. The official (BNF) tablets each contain either 10 or 20 mg of debrisoquine sulphate. The proprietary name is DECLINAX.

Guanoxan

guanoxan sulphate

Guanoxan is a very potent antihypertensive agent which produces noradrenergic neurone blockade together with a number of other pharmacological effects. It produces some reduction in the levels of catecholamines stored in the brain and the adrenal medullae as well as in peripheral sympathetic neurones. Unlike the other drugs in this class guanoxan reduces the sensitivity of peripheral tissues to catecholamines indicating that it has actions post-synaptically on adrenoreceptors as well as presynaptically on noradrenergic nerves. Despite its widespread effects it would appear that the important action of guanoxan in hypertension is noradrenergic neurone blockade.

Clinical use and dosage. In clinical use guanoxan has been shown to cause liver damage associated with jaundice in a number of patients. For this reason it is used solely to treat very severe hypertension refractory to other drugs. The starting oral dose is 10 mg daily which may be slowly increased up to 50 mg daily. Because of its tendency to cause liver damage it is advisable to perform regular tests of liver function in patients receiving it. It is available commercially (ENVACAR) in tablets of 10 and 40 mg strength.

Guanoclor

guanoclor sulphate

This is another substance which, like guanoxan, has a number of pharmacological actions in addition to noradrenergic neurone blockade. Like guanoxan it causes some depletion of both central and peripheral catecholamine stores which it may do partly by interfering with the conversion of dopamine to noradrenaline. Its onset of action is rather slow and a maximum effect occurs within 48 hours making adjustment of dosage more difficult than with bethanidine or debrisoquine.

Clinical uses and dosage. Guanoclor offers no advantages over better tried agents such as bethanidine and it tends to cause more gastrointestinal disturbance than either bethanidine or debrisoquine. The usual oral starting dose is 20 mg per day in divided doses and this may be gradually increased by 10 mg increments to give usual daily maintenance doses of 10 to 120 mg. Guanoclor has been shown to increase the plasma levels of some liver enzymes and it is therefore unwise to use it in patients with suspected liver disease. It is available commercially in tablets of 10 and 40 mg strength (VATENSOL).

GENERAL PRECAUTIONS ASSOCIATED WITH THE CLINICAL USE OF NORADRENERGIC NEURONE BLOCKERS

All the drugs of this class have a basically similar mode of action which is to interrupt transmission between sympathetic neurones and effector tissues of the cardiovascular system by preventing the release of noradrenaline from postganglionic sympathetic neurones. The fall in blood pressure which they produce is essentially orthostatic and their useful clinical action is therefore apparently inseparable from their most troublesome side-effects of producing postural and exertional hypotension. These drugs should be used cautiously in patients suffering from cerebrovascular or coronary artery disease since in these patients periods of profound hypotension may render perfusion of vital tissues inadequate and also provide conditions favouring thrombus formation. The problem of postural and exertional hypotension is most severe with guanethidine which, on account of its prolonged action, is particularly liable to cause hypotension on rising; it can be overcome partly by warning patients of the danger of sudden changes in either posture or the level of muscular work and also by using drugs with a briefer action such as bethanidine.

The noradrenergic neurone blockers, with the exception of guanoxan, have no blocking effects on adrenoreceptors in effector tissues and in addition they all have some inhibitory effect on the neuronal uptake process for catecholamines (Uptake$_1$). The result is that these substances produce a supersensitivity of the cardiovascular system to substances such as noradrenaline which are normally partly inactivated by the neuronal uptake mechanism. There is also evidence to suggest that these substances sensitise peripheral tissues to noradrenaline by a direct action on smooth muscle in addition to their inhibitory effects on Uptake$_1$. Consequently, patients receiving these drugs and requiring treatment with pressor drugs may require much lower doses of noradrenaline if undue cardiovascular stimulant effects are to be avoided. The supersensitivity to catecholamines induced by noradrenergic neurone blockers is also of consequence in the small number of hypertensive patients suffering from a tumour of the adrenal medulla (phaeochromocytoma) since these drugs do not prevent release of medullary catecholamines and by inhibiting Uptake$_1$ will potentiate the cardiovascular effects of circulating catecholamines. Phaeochromocytoma therefore constitutes an absolute contra-indication for noradrenergic neurone blockers.

It appears that noradrenergic neurone blockers are transported by Uptake$_1$ into the noradrenergic neurones where they produce their characteristic action on transmitter release. It follows that a number of drugs such as tricyclic antidepressants and amphetamine derivatives which themselves inhibit Uptake$_1$ are able to block the neuronal transport of noradrenergic neurone blockers and thus antagonise their antihypertensive action. This interaction will be discussed more fully later in this chapter. The noradrenergic neurone blockers cause bradycardia in most patients receiving them by abolishing sympathetic excitatory activity to the heart leading to a relative predominance of inhibitory vagal tone. It has been found that patients receiving these drugs who need to be anaesthetised for surgical procedures require an increased dose of atropine or hyoscine to provide protection of the heart from possible cardiac arrest. This potential hazard is most pronounced with guanethidine since its effects may persist in man for up to 3 weeks after discontinuing therapy. In clinical use all of the drugs in this class are liable to produce oedema as a result of sodium and water retention. The mechanism of this effect is not clear but it is readily reversed by small doses of thiazide diuretics which have the additional useful property of potentiating the antihypertensive effects of noradrenergic neurone blockers without increasing their side-effects resulting from sympathetic blockade.

It is particularly important that drugs used in the treatment of chronic conditions such as hypertension should be free from long-term toxic effects since they may need to be used for many years in some patients. In general, the noradrenergic neurone blockers, with the exception of guanoxan, have not produced any long-term toxic effects. Guanoxan has been shown to produce changes in liver function in a number of patients receiving it and for this reason its use should be restricted to the treatment of hypertensive crises or to patients in whom other antihypertensive drugs have been shown to be ineffective.

Mechanism of action of noradrenergic neurone blocking agents

Despite much research effort by a large number of workers the precise mechanism whereby these drugs induce failure of transmitter release in noradrenergic nerves is unknown. One suggestion that has been made for several of the drugs is that they interfere with the synthesis and/or storage of noradrenaline within sympathetic neurones. This suggestion originally arose because in isolated tissues high concentrations of TM10 were shown by Bain & Fielden (1957) to inhibit the conversion of dopamine to noradrenaline. However, it is doubtful whether this observation has any relevance to the action of the drug in preventing neuronal noradrenaline release in whole animals since the levels of TM10 in tissues after systemic administration are probably too low to significantly affect transmitter synthesis. It seems similarly unlikely that depletion of neuronal noradrenaline stores is the primary mechanism of action of these drugs. In animal experiments guanethidine is the most potent drug of this class in causing loss of neuronal noradrenaline although Cass & Spriggs (1961) showed that the onset of sympathetic blockade with this drug preceded any loss of transmitter from the nerves. Conversely, Day & Rand (1962) showed that after treatment of cats for up to a week with high doses of guanethidine full responses of the nictitating membrane to sympathetic stimulation could be produced by the administration of dexamphetamine which displaces guanethidine from neuronal storage sites (see Fig. 10.2). This experiment suggests that even when guanethidine has presumably produced its maximal noradrenaline depleting action sufficient noradrenaline remains for normal nerve function to occur. The evidence suggests that noradrenaline depletion may be a consequence of prolonged sympathetic blockade and not a direct cause of it. Supporting this concept is the finding that drugs such as TM10 and bretylium, whose

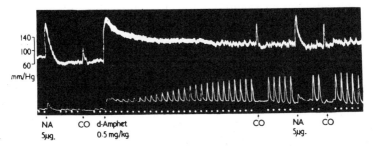

Fig. 10.2 Reversal of the noradrenergic neurone blocking action of guanethidine by dexamphetamine on the cat's nictitating membrane preparation. The cat in this experiment had been treated with daily doses of guanethidine (12.5 mg/Kg) for the 7 days prior to the experiment. Initially, the blood pressure was low and the responses to electrical stimulation of the sympathetic nerve to the nictitating membrane were almost absent and the reflex rise in blood pressure in response to occlusion of both carotid arteries (CO) was reduced. An intravenous injection of dexamphetamine (0·5 mg/Kg) restored the responses of the nictitating membrane to sympathetic stimulation, increased the basal level of arterial blood pressure and increased the pressor response to bilateral carotid artery occlusion. (From Day & Rand, 1962).

short-term sympathetic blocking actions are not associated with noradrenaline depletion, may produce depletion after prolonged periods of treatment with full blocking doses.

An early theory to explain the mode of action of these drugs was that by virtue of their local anaesthetic activity they blocked conduction in the fine non-myelinated postganglionic sympathetic neurones. This theory is supported by the fact that all the compounds currently in use have local anaesthetic activity and by the observation of Boura, Copp, Duncombe, Green & McCoubrey (1960) that bretylium is accumulated by noradrenergic neurones to produce local concentrations similar to those which if applied to the outside of the nerves interfered with conduction of action potentials. However, Exley (1957) showed that in concentrations sufficient to block sympathetic nerve responses TM10 did not impair conduction of action potentials in the same nerve. Moreover he was unable to show any correlation between local anaesthetic activity and ability to block sympathetic nerve responses in the TM10 series of compounds. It is not possible to totally discount the local anaesthetic hypothesis since it has been argued that the point at which nerve conduction may be impaired by noradrenergic neurone blocking agents is the very fine terminal varicosities and not the nerve trunks of sympathetic nerves. The outcome of this particular debate will have to await the development of more sophisticated techniques for examining the electrophysiological events in terminal varicosities of sympathetic nerves.

Burn & Rand (1960) suggested that noradrenergic neurone blockers may act by preventing the action of acetylcholine in releasing noradrenaline in the 'cholinergic link' mechanism which they have postulated operates in noradrenergic nerves. The hypothesis is an attractive one and most of the noradrenergic neurone blockers tested do have weak anti-acetylcholine actions. However, there has been little experimental evidence to support the idea.

It would seem that whatever the precise mechanism of action of these drugs in preventing noradrenaline release it is very likely that they exert this action intraneuronally. Thus there is a great deal of evidence which suggests that these compounds are transported by Uptake$_1$ to the inside of noradrenergic neurones. It has been shown that when Uptake$_1$ is inhibited by drugs such as the tricyclic antidepressants or by indirectly acting sympathomimetics such as dexamphetamine then both the intraneuronal accumulation of the noradrenergic neurone blockers and their sympathetic blocking action are prevented. The fact that all the noradrenergic neurone blockers in clinical use are antagonised in this way suggests that they are all transported by Uptake$_1$ and that they may produce their effects on noradrenergic neurones by a basically similar mechanism. Once inside the neurone most of the drugs in this class cause some initial displacement of stored noradrenaline by a mechanism apparently similar to that of indirectly-acting sympathomimetic amines. This initial sympathomimetic effect of noradrenergic neurone blockers does not appear to be directly related to the slow depletion of neuronal noradrenaline which agents such as guanethidine produce on long-term treatment. There is also evidence to suggest that after guanethidine blockade of sympathetic responses then small amounts of the drug are released by nerve impulses by an apparently similar mechanism to that by which noradrenaline is normally released. The significance of this observation is unclear but it would seem unlikely that guanethidine could take over the transmitter role of noradrenaline in the way that α-methylnoradrenaline formed from α-methyldopa is believed to do (see Chapter 13).

A possible explanation for the intraneuronal effects of these drugs is that they in some way stabilise the membrane of the noradrenaline storage vesicles such that the vesicles can no longer extrude their contents into the synaptic cleft on passage of nerve impulses. Such a mechanism might explain several of the properties which these compounds have in common such as local anaesthetic activity and a tendency to inhibit transmitter synthesis and storage.

Interaction of noradrenergic neurone blockers with drugs which inhibit Uptake₁

As mentioned previously drugs which inhibit $Uptake_1$ antagonise the action of noradrenergic neurone blocking drugs. Day & Rand (1963) showed that the antagonism between dexamphetamine and guanethidine had many of the characteristics of a competitive antagonism. Drugs which inhibit $Uptake_1$ include cocaine, tricyclic antidepressants such as desipramine and amitryptyline, and also dexamphetamine and related substances such as ephedrine, mephentermine and methylphenidate. Indirectly-acting sympathomimetics such as dexamphetamine which are immune to destruction by monoamine oxidase in addition to preventing the action of subsequently administered noradrenergic neurone blockers are also able to reverse the blocking action of these substances once established (see Fig. 10.2). On the other hand, substances such as desipramine which inhibit $Uptake_1$ but do not themselves produce sympathomimetic effects, are effective at preventing the onset of noradrenergic neurone blockade but rather less effective in reversing a block once established. The explanation of this difference is that indirectly-acting sympathomimetics appear to actually displace noradrenergic neurone blockers from intraneuronal sites as well as preventing their uptake.

The antagonism between drugs which inhibit $Uptake_1$ and noradrenergic neurone blockers is of clinical significance since tricyclic antidepressants and amphetamine derivatives with anorexic properties have been used in hypertensive patients receiving drugs such as guanethidine and bethanidine with a resultant loss of the antihypertensive effect (see Fig. 10.3). It is possible that some of the cases of reported tolerance in patients receiving noradrenergic neurone blocking agents may have in fact been due to pharmacological antagonism by concurrently administered drugs.

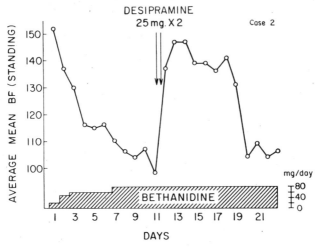

Fig. 10.3 Antagonism of the antihypertensive action of bethanidine by desipramine in a hypertensive patient. The dose of bethanidine was adjusted by increments to 80 mg per day which produced a fall in standing mean blood pressure of about 50 mm Hg. The administration of two 25 mg tablets of desipramine prevented the blood pressure lowering action of bethanidine for approximately a week. (From Mitchell *et al.*, 1967).

SUMMARY

The noradrenergic neurone blocking drugs impair the functioning of peripheral sympathetic nerves by selectively preventing the release of noradrenaline from postganglionic noradrenergic neurones. They do not, in general, block adrenoreceptors in effector tissues nor do they impair responses to stimulation of either parasympathetic or sympathetic cholinergic nerves or the release of catecholamines from the adrenal medullae. They were formerly much used in the treatment of hypertension since their lack of effect on the parasympathetic system gave them significant clinical advantages over the ganglion blocking agents. At the present time their clinical use is mainly restricted to patients suffering from severe hypertension or to patients who are unresponsive to milder antihypertensive drugs. In man these agents lower arterial blood pressure by lowering peripheral resistance by inhibiting vasoconstrictor sympathetic tone and also by reducing cardiac output by reducing venous return.

The prototype of this group of drugs was xylocholine (TM10) which was not used clinically because it possessed a variety of acetylcholine-like effects. Bretylium was the first drug of this type to be used in man but its clinical use was limited because most patients became tolerant to its effects. Guanethidine superseded bretylium in clinical use and has been the most clinically used drug of this class. It is more potent than bretylium, has a longer duration of action and patients much less frequently become tolerant to its effects. The major disadvantages of guanethidine are that it causes postural and exertional hypotension and diarrhoea in many patients receiving it. Bethanidine and debrisoquine are later drugs of this class which have a briefer duration of action than guanethidine, are easier to use clinically and have a reduced tendency to cause diarrhoea.

The precise mechanism whereby these drugs produce their effects on noradrenergic nerves is not clear but the evidence suggests that their main site of action is intraneuronal. Drugs such as tricyclic antidepressants and amphetamine derivatives which impair the noradrenergic neuronal catecholamine uptake mechanism (Uptake$_1$) prevent both the intraneuronal accumulation of noradrenergic neurone blockers and also their inhibitory action on noradrenaline release.

REFERENCES

Bain, W. A. & Fielden, R. (1957) In-vitro formation of noradrenaline from dopamine by human tissue. *Lancet*, **2**, 472–473.

Boura, A. L. A. & Green, A. F. (1959) The actions of bretylium, adrenergic neurone blocking and other effects. *Br. J. Pharmac.*, **14**, 536–548.

Boura, A. L. A., Copp, F. C., Duncombe, W. G., Green, A. F. & McCoubrey, A. (1960) The selective accumulation of bretylium in sympathetic ganglia and their postganglionic nerves. *Br. J. Pharmac.*, **15**, 265–270.

Bron, A. J. (1969) Sympathetic control of aqueous secretion in man. *Br. J. Ophthal.*, **53**, 37–45.

Burn, J. H. & Rand, M. J. (1960) Sympathetic postganglionic cholinergic fibres. *Br. J. Pharmac.*, **15**, 56–66.

Cass, R. & Spriggs, T. L. B. (1961) Tissue amine levels and sympathetic blockade after guanethidine and bretylium. *Br. J. Pharmac.*, **17**, 442–450.

Day, M. D. & Rand, M. J. (1962) Antagonism of guanethidine by dexamphetamine and other related sympathomimetic amines. *J. Pharm. Pharmac.*, **14**, 541–549.

Day, M. D. & Rand, M. J. (1963) Evidence for a competitive antagonism of guanethidine by dexamphetamine. *Br. J. Pharmac.*, **20**, 17–28.

Exley, K. A. (1957) The blocking action of choline 2:6 xylyl ether bromide on adrenergic nerves. *Br. J. Pharmac.*, **12**, 297–305.

Hey, P. & Willey, G. L. (1954) Choline 2:6 xylyl ether bromide; an active quaternary local anaesthetic. *Br. J. Pharmac.*, **9**, 471–475.

Maxwell, R. A., Mull, R. P. & Plummer, A. J. (1959) [2-(octahydro-1-azocinyl)-ethyl]-guanidine sulfate (CIBA 5864-SU), a new synthetic antihypertensive agent. *Experientia*, **15**, 267.

Mitchell, J. R., Arias, L. & Oates, J. A. (1967) Antagonism of the antihypertensive action of guanethidine sulfate by desipramine hydrochloride. *J.A.M.A.*, **202**, 973–976.

GENERAL READING

Boura, A. L. A. & Green, A. F. (1965) Adrenergic neurone blocking agents. *A. Rev. Pharmac.*, **5**, 183–212.

Copp, F. C. (1964) Adrenergic neurone blocking agents. *Adv. Drug Res.*, **1**, 161–189.

Furst, C. I. (1967) The Biochemistry of Guanethidine. *Adv. Drug Res.*, **4**, 133–161.

11

α-Adrenoreceptor blocking agents

The basic classification of adrenoreceptors into α and β types was discussed in Chapters 8 and 9. The present chapter deals with the pharmacology and therapeutic uses of substances whose main action is to combine with α-adrenoreceptors and in so doing to prevent their activation by sympathomimetics including catecholamines released from sympathetic nerves and from the adrenal medullae. Most of the important pharmacological effects of these compounds are explained by their actions in blocking post-synaptic α-adrenoreceptors. However, in common with other post-synaptic blocking agents, such as the antimuscarinics (see Chapter 6), they are relatively more effective in blocking the effects of exogenously administered agonists than in blocking the responses to transmitter released endogenously from nerves. Possible explanations of this phenomenon have already been discussed for the antimuscarinics (see pages 71–72) and a further explanation in the case of the α-adreno-receptor blocking agents is afforded by the ability of most of them to increase noradrenaline release from noradrenergic nerves by a presynaptic action; this effect will be discussed more fully later in the present chapter.

The selective inhibition of some of the physiological effects of both adrenaline and sympathetic stimulation was first reported as early as 1906. In that year Dale demonstrated that extracts of ergot, a fungus which may infect rye, changed the usual blood pressure responses of the anaesthetised cat to both intravenously administered adrenaline and electrical stimulation of the splanchnic nerve from rises to falls in blood pressure. The classification of adrenoreceptors into α and β types by Ahlquist (1948) afforded an explanation of these observations since all the effects of adrenaline and sympathetic stimulation blocked by ergot alkaloids are in fact effects produced by stimulation of α-adrenoreceptors. Later work has led to the synthesis of a very large number of compounds with the ability to more or less

selectively antagonise the effects of α-adrenoreceptor stimulation. Most of these compounds block α-adrenoreceptors by
competition with α-agonists for the receptor sites and thus the
degree of blockade obtained is related to the relative concentrations of agonist and antagonist present. However, one group of
α-adrenoreceptor antagonists, the haloalkylamines, produce a
non-competitive antagonism which cannot be overcome by
increasing the concentration of α-agonist present. This type of
compound produces a very prolonged blocking action which is
sometimes referred to as 'irreversible' or 'insurmountable'.

In general, the α-adrenoreceptor blocking drugs have been of
considerable experimental value in uncovering the complexities
of the autonomic nervous system but have proved to be of only
limited clinical usefulness. Undoubtedly much of the interest in
this group of compounds was due to the hope that they would
be of value in the treatment of hypertension. However, despite
the antagonism of the vasoconstrictor effects of α-adrenoreceptor stimulants and of sympathetic stimulation which they
cause and which results in dilatation of peripheral blood vessels,
their effectiveness in lowering arterial blood pressure is limited
by the marked increase in sympathetic nerve activity to the
myocardium which they produce and which is at least partly
reflex in origin. Cardiac adrenoreceptors being predominantly
of the β-type are unaffected by α-adrenoreceptor antagonists and
thus tachycardia and increased cardiac output result from the
lowering of peripheral vascular resistance which they produce.
In the treatment of essential hypertension noradrenergic neurone
blocking agents such as bethanidine (see Chapter 10) are generally more effective than the α-adrenoreceptor blockers since
the former drugs prevent the release of transmitter from noradrenergic nerves in tissues containing α and/or β-adrenoreceptors. Despite their lack of established usefulness in most
forms of hypertension the α-adrenoreceptor antagonists are
mainly used clinically for their ability to produce vasodilatation
which makes them of some use in the treatment of vascular
disorders characterised by excessive vasoconstriction. Their
other clinical uses are based on their action in antagonising many
of the actions of circulating sympathomimetic substances which
renders them of use in the diagnosis and treatment of phaeochromocytoma and in the emergency treatment of hypertensive
crises due to overdosage with sympathomimetic substances.

As a class the α-adrenoreceptor blockers tend to be somewhat
less specific in their pharmacological actions than, for instance,

the β-adrenoreceptor blockers and some α-adrenoreceptor antagonists may modify responses to other substances such as acetylcholine, histamine and 5-HT. It is possible that some part of the therapeutic actions of α-adrenoreceptor blockers are due to these and other actions rather than to specific blockade of α-adrenoreceptors.

α-ADRENORECEPTOR BLOCKERS IN CLINICAL USE

Ergot alkaloids

As mentioned previously ergot is a fungus which may infect rye and which historically has been responsible for a number of outbreaks of poisoning with a characteristic spectrum of symptoms (*ergotism*) and usually caused by the eating of bread made from infected rye. Ergot contains twelve alkaloids (six isomeric pairs) of complex chemical structure and each derived from lysergic acid amide. The two major actions of ergot alkaloids are to stimulate smooth muscle and to block α-adrenoreceptors. *Ergotamine* is an important ergot alkaloid and possesses both of these properties producing both vasoconstriction and α-adrenoreceptor blockade; it is used clinically in the treatment of migraine. Dihydrogenation of the lysergic acid nucleus of ergotamine and of the other ergot alkaloids increases α-adrenoreceptor blocking potency but reduces smooth muscle stimulant activity. *Dihydroergotamine* is also used to treat migraine. *Ergometrine* is an alkaloid with only feeble effects in blocking α-adrenoreceptors but with a powerful action in stimulating smooth muscle especially that of the uterus (*oxytocic action*); it is extensively used in obstetrics to reduce post-partum bleeding which it does mainly by contracting the uterus.

Ergotoxine was the name given to the first alkaloidal fraction isolated from ergot and used by Dale (1906) in his classic experiments. For many years ergotoxine was thought to be a single substance but later work showed it to be a mixture of three different alkaloids *ergocornine, ergocristine* and *ergocryptine* (Fig. 11.1). Ergotoxine has α-adrenoreceptor blocking activity and in addition stimulates the smooth muscle of blood vessels and the uterus. However, the dihydroderivatives of the mixture have increased potency in blocking α-adrenoreceptors and very little smooth muscle stimulant activity.

Clinical uses and dosage of dihydroergotoxine. The preparation of dihydroergotoxine which is used clinically is a mixture containing equal parts of the methane sulphonate salts of dihydroergocornine, dihydroergocristine and dihydroergocryptine (proprietary name HYDERGINE). It has been used to cause peripheral vasodilatation in occlusive vascular conditions such as Raynaud's syndrome. It has little effect on the blood pressure of normotensive individuals but may lower it in hypertensive patients. It is probable that a central action reducing sympathetic efferent nerve activity contributes to both its blood pressure lowering and vasodilating activities. It is rather poorly absorbed

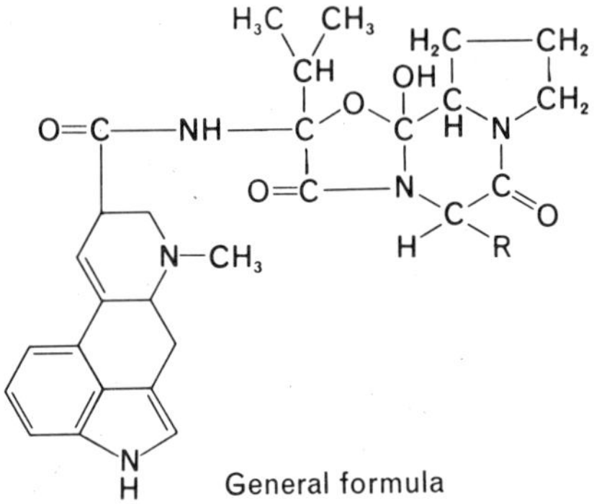

General formula

Ergocornine R = —CH(CH$_3$)$_2$

Ergocristine R = —CH$_2$—⬡—

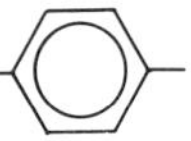

Ergocryptine R = —CH$_2$·CH(CH$_3$)$_2$

Fig. 11.1 Structural formulae of ergot alkaloids with α-adrenoreceptor antagonist activity; a mixture of the above three compounds is known as ergotoxine.

by mouth but may be given sub-lingually in doses of up to 4·5 mg per day in the form of tablets each containing a total of 1·5 mg of the alkaloids in equal proportions. It has also been administered by intramuscular or intra-arterial injection in doses of 150 to 600 micrograms to relieve vascular spasm.

In recent years several reports have appeared which suggest that dihydroergotoxine may improve the mental status of elderly patients showing signs of inadequate cerebral blood flow. Such actions are difficult to quantify and it has been suggested, but with little supporting evidence, that the beneficial effects are due to increased cerebral blood flow.

The mechanism of action of the ergot alkaloids in relieving migraine is not known. It was thought at one time that the effect was due to constriction of cerebral blood vessels since migraine attacks are associated with cerebral vasodilatation and ergota-mine is a potent vasoconstrictor. However, it is likely that the mechanism is more complex than this since dihydroergotamine has a reduced vasoconstrictor action but retains its anti-migraine action.

The clinical use of dihydroergotoxine and the other ergot alkaloids are limited by their tendency to cause nausea and vomiting as well as other side-effects such as blurred vision, skin rashes and nasal stuffiness.

Tolazoline hydrochloride BP

This substance is a derivative of imidazoline and is structurally related to α-adrenoreceptor stimulants such as xylometazoline (Chapter 9) and clonidine (Chapter 13). It is a competitive antagonist of α-adrenoreceptors but has a number of other pharmacological actions. For instance, it has an action resembling that of histamine in stimulating gastric acid secretion and another resembling acetylcholine in stimulating gastrointestinal motility. In the usual doses used in man tolazoline produces only weak blockade of α-adrenoreceptors and it is likely that a considerable part of its vasodilator activity is due to direct effects on vascular smooth muscle possibly related to its actions in stimulating histamine and acetylcholine receptors. In man, tolazoline increases venous capacity, decreases peripheral resistance yet produces little effect on the level of arterial blood pressure since cardiac output is increased. The increased cardiac output is partly due to a reflex increase in cardiac sympathetic nerve activity consequent on the fall in blood pressure and probably partly due to an increase in release of noradrenaline from noradrenergic nerves caused by a presynaptic action of the drug (see later in this chapter).

Clinical uses and dosage. Tolazoline is well absorbed after oral administration and is mostly excreted unchanged in the urine. It is used in man to increase peripheral blood flow in vaso-spastic conditions such as Raynaud's syndrome, chilblains and intermittent claudication. It has also been used to increase the blood flow through recently grafted tissues after plastic surgery. It is used in man in oral daily doses of up to 200 mg administered in divided doses. Its maximum effects after oral administration is attained in 45 to 100 minutes and its effects persist for several hours. Its onset of action is quicker if administered by the intramuscular route and it has also been administered intravenously or intra-arterially in the treatment of severe arterial spasm such as may occur in cases of gangrene. The usual parenteral dose of the drug is 50 mg and injections are sometimes given to assess the likely benefit to be gained from sympathectomy. The cardiac stimulant actions of tolazoline have precipitated cardiac arrhythmias in some patients and it is used with extreme caution in patients suffering from cardiac disease. Its action in stimulating gastric acid secretion precludes its use in patients suffering from gastric or peptic ulceration. The official (BP) tablets of tolazoline hydrochloride contain 25 mg of active ingredient and a similar preparation is available under the proprietary name of PRISCOL.

Phentolamine Mesylate BP

Phentolamine is also derived from imidazoline but it is a more potent α-adrenoreceptor antagonist and has a somewhat narrower spectrum of other pharmacological activity than tolazoline. However, like tolazoline, it appears that at least part of its vasodilator activity in man is due to direct action on blood vessels rather than to specific blockade of α-adrenoreceptors. Phentolamine in usual doses used in man often causes some lowering of arterial blood pressure and this may be associated with postural hypotension. The other side-effects of phentolamine resemble those of tolazoline except that it does not provoke the secretion of gastric acid.

Clinical uses and dosage. Phentolamine is poorly absorbed orally and is usually administered intravenously and occasionally intramuscularly. At one time phentolamine was widely used, especially in the USA, in the diagnosis of phaeochromocytoma. In this condition paroxysmal bouts of hypertension occur as a result of secretion of excessive amounts of catecholamines from a tumour of adrenal medullary cells. Intravenous phentolamine (usual dose 5 mg) produces a fall of arterial blood pressure of at least 35 mm Hg systolic and 25 mm Hg diastolic within two minutes in most patients suffering from phaeochromocytoma but not usually in patients suffering from other types of secondary or from primary (essential) hypertension. The test has proved helpful in the past in providing a rapid clue as to the cause of hypertension but it may give occasional false positive results in patients suffering from uraemia and also in those who have taken sedatives or narcotics in the 24 hours before the test. False negative results, although less common, have occurred in patients with a tumour which was insufficiently secreting at the time of the test or where the effects of the phaeochromocytoma are partly obscured by the simultaneous presence of essential hypertension. With the advent of chemical methods for the estimation of catecholamines and their metabolites in urine the phentolamine test for the diagnosis of phaeochromocytoma has declined in importance. Intravenous or intramuscular doses of phentolamine (5 to 10 mg) may be given preoperatively to patients undergoing surgery for removal of a phaeochromocytoma in order to prevent the large fluctuations in blood pressure which may occur during the surgical handling of the tumour.

Possibly the most important uses for phentolamine at the present time are as an antidote to the pressor effects of overdoses of α-adrenoreceptor stimulant substances and in the treatment of hypertensive crises such as those which may result from the interaction of some sympathomimetics or naturally occurring amines with monoamine oxidase inhibiting drugs (see Chapter 9).

Phentolamine is officially (BP) available as an injection containing 10 mg of the methane sulphonate in one ml and as a similar proprietary preparation (ROGITINE).

Phenoxybenzamine hydrochloride BP

This substance is one of a group of compounds, the haloalkylamines, of which more than 1,500 have been synthesised and tested experimentally since the first member of the series, dibenamine, was described by Nickerson & Goodman in 1947. Of these compounds phenoxybenzamine is the only one in clinical use at the present time. It is a potent α-adrenoreceptor antagonist with a slow onset but prolonged duration of action. In common with other α-adrenoreceptor blockers phenoxy-benzamine has a number of other pharmacological actions including antagonism of acetylcholine, histamine and 5-HT receptors. However, it appears that the vasodilator actions of the drug in man are essentially due to α-adrenoreceptor blockade

negatively charged
site on α-adrenoreceptor

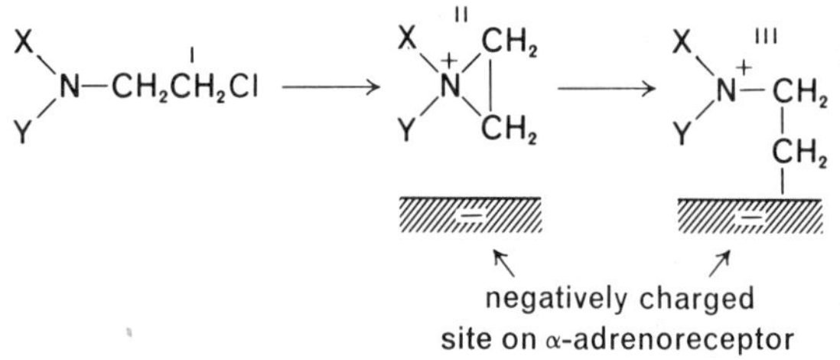

Fig. 11.2 Combination of phenoxybenzamine with α-adrenoreceptor; in I unchanged molecule of phenoxybenzamine in II the molecule has undergone cyclisation to form an ethylene imminium ion which is attached to the α-adrenoreceptor by electrostatic forces to produce competitive inhibition; in III by molecular rearrangement the antagonist has alkylated the α-adrenoreceptor via formation of a covalent bond to produce an irreversible antagonism.

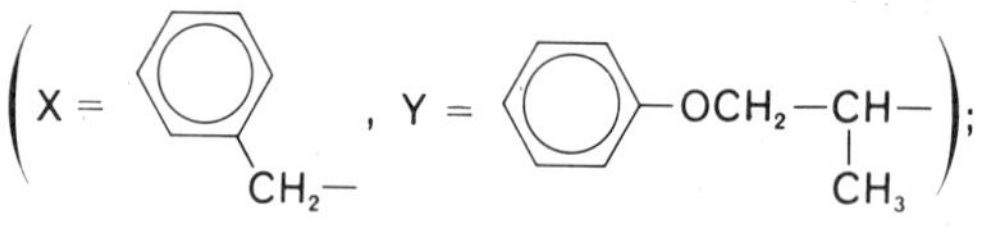

and it does not have any direct relaxant action on vascular smooth muscle. The slow onset of action of phenoxybenzamine is due to the formation of an intermediate compound which is the active species of the drug. The intermediate compound forms an ethylene imminium ion (see Fig. 11.2) which is believed to attach to a negatively-charged site on the α-receptor. Molecular rearrangement then occurs which results in the α-site being alkylated via formation of a covalent chemical bond with the antagonist. The covalent bond formed is much stronger than the ionic bond formed by either α-adrenoreceptor agonists or competitive antagonists and explains both the prolonged duration of phenoxybenzamine's action and the fact that it cannot be readily reversed by α-adrenoreceptor agonists. The early stage of the α-adrenoreceptor blockade produced by phenoxybenzamine is apparently competitive in nature since it can be overcome by α-adrenoreceptor agonists or be prevented by 'protection' of the α-adrenoreceptors by prior treatment with competitive α-adrenoreceptor antagonists. However, once the blockade has fully developed it cannot be overcome by either treatment. The irreversible nature of the blockade of α-adreno-receptors by the haloalkylamines has made them valuable research tools to physiologists and pharmacologists in uncovering autonomic mechanisms.

The general effects of phenoxybenzamine in man are similar to those already described for the other α-adrenoreceptor antagonists, the main difference being its slow onset and more prolonged duration of action. In man the full effect of an intra-venous dose of phenoxybenzamine take up to an hour to become fully effective and, once established, signs of α-adrenoreceptor blockade may persist for 3-4 days. In normotensive patients phenoxybenzamine produces variable effects on resting arterial blood pressure but interferes with reflex adjustments of pressure producing marked postural hypotension. In hypertensive patients and in persons with a reduced blood volume it may produce quite marked reductions in blood pressure. In common with other antagonists of α-adrenoreceptors phenoxybenzamine causes a marked increase in cardiac output due partly to reflex effects and also to presynaptic effects on the cardiac sympathetic nerves leading to an increased output of noradrenaline and also to a delay in its inactivation. Phenoxybenzamine has an effect in antagonising cardiac arrhythmias provoked by catecholamines and this has led to the suggestion that myocardial α-adreno-receptors may be involved in the genesis of such irregularities of cardiac rhythm. There is considerable evidence that phenoxy-benzamine penetrates into the brain after oral administration and it may give rise to central effects such as hyperventilation, motor excitability and feelings of nausea. Some patients taking the drug also experience feelings of tiredness and lethargy. It is not clear which, if any, of these central actions are due to α-adrenoreceptor blockade.

Clinical uses and dosage. Although it is incompletely absorbed by the oral route phenoxybenzamine is most often given by mouth in daily commencing doses of 10 mg which may be increased gradually up to a daily maximum of about 240 mg. The drug has also been used intravenously in doses of 0·5 to 1 mg/kg; it is too irritant for other parenteral routes of ad-ministration. Phenoxybenzamine is used to treat a variety of

vasospastic conditions including Raynaud's disease and intermittent claudication. It has been successfully used in the long-
term treatment of inoperable phaeochromocytoma and also to
provide prolonged α-adrenoreceptor blockade before surgical
removal of adrenal medullary tumours.

An apparently paradoxical use which has been suggested for
phenoxybenzamine and other α-adrenoreceptor antagonists is
in the treatment of shock syndromes associated with hypotension. The rationale for this treatment is that these conditions
are often associated with profound constriction of some vascular
beds which may lead to insufficient blood perfusion of some vital
tissues. It is argued that in such patients the use of a vasodilator
together with appropriate intravenous fluid replacement will
restore tissue perfusion and aid recovery. The treatment has
been reported to be strikingly effective in some patients but much
less so in others and as yet there is no way of predicting which
patients are likely to be benefitted. The treatment is of potential
danger if instituted in hypovolaemic patients since it may cause
a further reduction in venous return and hence cardiac output.

It has been reported that small doses of phenoxybenzamine are
effective in restoring the sensitivity to the action of noradrenergic
neurone blocking agents in patients who have become refractory
to them. A recent use for phenoxybenzamine which has been
claimed is the treatment of *anorexia nervosa*. This condition is
associated with a marked reduction in body weight due to a
psychological aversion to food. It remains to be seen whether
this report will be confirmed by subsequent studies and also
whether the effect is due to antagonism of central α-adrenoreceptors. Phenoxybenzamine is available commercially in the
form of capsules each containing 10 mg of the active principle
(proprietary name DIBENYLINE).

Thymoxamine hydrochloride

Thymoxamine is a competitive and relatively selective α-
adrenoreceptor antagonist. Apart from weak antihistaminic
activity it appears that all its useful effects in man are attributable

to blockade of α-adrenoreceptors. It is well absorbed by mouth and has a duration of action of 3 to 4 hours.

Clinical uses and dosage. The clinical uses of thymoxamine are similar to those described for the other drugs of this class. The recommended oral adult dose is 40 mg repeated 4 times daily. In usual clinical doses it has little effect on blood pressure but it occasionally causes mild diarrhoea, nausea and/or headache in some patients. It is also used by subcutaneous, intramuscular or intra-arterial routes in the treatment of vasospastic conditions. The relative specificity of its actions and its moderate duration of action make it useful for assessing the likely outcome of surgical sympathectomy. It is commercially available as tablets each containing 40 mg of thymoxamine base (OPILON TAB-LETS) and as injections containing either 5 mg of base in each 1 ml ampoule (OPILON AMPOULES) or 30 mg of base in 2 ml ampoules (OPILON FORTE).

Prazosin hydrochloride

Prazosin is a recently introduced drug with vasodilator activity and found to be of value in the treatment of hypertension. It was at first thought that the drug acted predominantly by a direct relaxant action on vascular smooth muscle but subsequent studies have indicated that it has additional potent α-adreno-receptor antagonist activity. The haemodynamic effects of prazosin in man differ in important respects from those of other α-adrenoreceptor antagonists such as phenoxybenzamine. Thus prazosin produces much less postural hypotension than other α-adrenoreceptor antagonists and its blood pressure lowering effect is not accompanied by any significant increase in heart rate. These beneficial effects are believed to be due firstly to its vasodilator action being exerted mainly on arterioles so that peripheral resistance is reduced without a marked reduction in venous return to the heart and secondly to the fact that prazosin does not appear to share the property of other α-adrenoreceptor antagonists of increasing noradrenaline output from sympathetic nerves by a presynaptic mechanism.

Clinical use and dosage. Although the drug has thus far only received limited clinical usage it is apparently a potent and effective antihypertensive agent. The side-effects of the drug generally appear to be mild apart from profound hypotension often accompanied by loss of consciousness which may occur in a few sensitive patients particularly at the beginning of treatment. The drug is used in commencing doses of 2 mg repeated three times daily which after a period of 4 to 6 weeks may be adjusted to maintenance doses of 3 to 20 mg daily in divided doses. Prazosin has been given concurrently with other antihypertensives such as β-adrenoreceptor antagonists and thiazide diuretics with good results. The drug is available commercially as tablets of either 2 or 5 mg strength under the trade-names of HYPOVASE and SINETINS.

Other α-adrenoreceptor antagonists

Many α-adrenoreceptor antagonists have been tested clinically but only the few already described in this chapter are at present used clinically in the United Kingdom. The *benzodioxans* are a group of compounds which have been extensively studied largely as a result of the efforts of the French chemist Fourneau. The only compound of the series to be commonly used clinically was *piperoxan* which produced a relatively transient competitive blockade. Piperoxan is not particularly specific for α-adrenoreceptors and produces a large number of other actions in the body. It is very much more effective in blocking responses to circulating α-agonists than against the effects of sympathetic stimulation. It is no longer used clinically in the United Kingdom.

Yohimbine is a plant alkaloid which is an indolealkylamine derivative chemically related to reserpine (Chapter 13). It produces a short-acting competitive blockade of α-adrenoreceptors and has in addition a wide spectrum of other actions including marked stimulation of the brain and reputed aphrodisiac properties. It is not used clinically as an α-adrenoreceptor antagonist.

Azapetine is a synthetic substance with both α-adrenoreceptor blocking and direct vasodilator actions closely resembling those of tolazoline. It is used clinically in the USA.

General comments on the clinical use of α-adrenoreceptor blocking drugs

A large amount of scientific effort has gone into the synthesis and testing of this group of drugs and it must be said that this endeavour has not been fully repaid by their clinical usefulness. The α-adrenoreceptor blocking agents have been repeatedly tested clinically for their antihypertensive effects but apart from some use in the diagnosis and treatment of phaeochromocytoma they have been found to be generally disappointing in the treatment of essential hypertension. The lack of useful effect of these drugs in hypertensive patients appears to be at least partly due to the cardiac stimulation and increase in cardiac output which most of them provoke. There have been some clinical reports of the cardiac effects of α-adrenoreceptor blockade being successfully overcome by concurrent treatment with a β-adrenoreceptor antagonist. This idea has been taken a stage further by the introduction into therapy of a single compound, labetalol (see Chapter 12), possessing both α and β-adrenoreceptor antagonist activity. In addition, the recently introduced drug prazosin produces α-adrenoreceptor blockade without significant reflex cardiac stimulant effects.

The place of α-adrenoreceptor antagonists in the treatment of peripheral vascular disorders is also somewhat insecure. The British National Formulary (1976–1978) states, 'The hope that these (α-adrenoreceptor antagonists) might help patients with vasospasm such as Raynaud's syndrome has not been realised.' This is an extreme viewpoint not fully confirmed by many clinical reports. Much confusion has been caused by the use of these drugs in patients suffering from occlusive vascular disorders associated with marked degenerative changes such as atherosclerosis in which pharmacological agents are unable to improve blood flow because of the mechanical state of the vessels. In some patients similar lack of success has been experienced using other vasodilator drugs such as muscarinic receptor and β-adrenoreceptor agonists. There is a considerable amount of evidence to suggest that α-adrenoreceptor antagonists are of value in the treatment of vasoconstriction caused by an increased sensitivity to sympathetic stimuli and to circulating catecholamines and in conditions where skin blood flow is impaired. Thus these drugs appear to be of help in the treatment of chilblains, cold extremities and ischaemic skin ulcers.

The reports of the beneficial effects on the mental status of elderly patients following treatment with vasodilator drugs such as dihydroergotoxine are of great interest but await convincing confirmation in carefully controlled trials as does the use of α-adrenoreceptor antagonists in the treatment of hypotensive states.

The most clear-cut clinical indications for the use of α-adrenoreceptor blockers is to antagonise the vasoconstrictor effects of circulating sympathomimetic substances arising either from a phaeochromocytoma or as a result of overdosage with sympathomimetic drugs.

Presynaptic actions of α-adrenoreceptor antagonists

Brown & Gillespie (1957) reported that the amount of noradrenaline appearing in the venous blood leaving the cat spleen after sympathetic stimulation was markedly increased after phenoxybenzamine. The interpretation of this observation was complicated by the later findings that phenoxybenzamine inhibits both the specific neuronal catecholamine uptake mechanism (Uptake$_1$) and the extraneuronal uptake mechanism (Uptake$_2$). However, by the use of other α-adrenoreceptor antagonists in appropriate concentrations many later workers have shown that these drugs increase the release per impulse of noradrenaline from sympathetic nerves by blocking presynaptic α-adrenoreceptors whose normal function is to be stimulated by neuronally released noradrenaline and to reduce the further output of noradrenaline. This negative feed-back loop is particularly effective at low rates of impulse traffic in sympathetic nerves. The mechanism whereby activation of presynaptic α-adrenoreceptors inhibits neuronal noradrenaline release is not clear but appears to involve a reduction in availability of intraneuronal calcium ions which are necessary for release of transmitter by nerve impulses. The release of intraneuronal noradrenaline by the indirectly-acting sympathomimetic substance tyramine is not dependent on calcium ions and is not reduced by stimulation of presynaptic α-adrenoreceptors. At high rates of impulse flow it is likely that a surplus of calcium ions are available for use by the transmitter release mechanism and hence presynaptic inhibition is relatively ineffective under these conditions.

The findings of presynaptic inhibitory α-adrenoreceptors is of considerable experimental interest and may also have some implications for the clinical use of both α-adrenoreceptor agonists and antagonists. For instance, the mechanism affords at least a partial explanation for the marked cardiac stimulation caused by some α-antagonists as well as for the sometimes very great differences in their activity against circulating catecholamines compared with the effects against noradrenaline released from nerves. In both cases increased release of neuronal noradrenaline induced by blockade of presynaptic α-adrenoreceptors would account for the observed effects.

Recent work (see review by Starke, 1977) indicates that pre- and postsynaptic α-adrenoreceptors may not be identical since agonists and antagonists of α-adrenoreceptors have been shown to have differing selectivities for each. Thus the α-agonists xylometazoline (Chapter 9) and clonidine (Chapter 13) have preferential effects on presynaptic α-adrenoreceptors whilst phenylephrine and methoxamine are selective for postsynaptic receptors. Noradrenaline itself is equiactive on pre- and post-synaptic receptors. The activity of some α-adrenoreceptor antagonists is similarly selective since tolazoline, piperoxan and yohimbine are selective for presynaptic receptors whilst thymoxamine and prazosin are selective for postsynaptic receptors.

Although the significance of presynaptic α-adrenoreceptors in the physiological release of noradrenaline from sympathetic nerves is not clear, it is possible that the search for more selective agonists and antagonists of pre- and postsynaptic adreno-receptors will lead to a further understanding of the function of these receptors and hopefully also to the production of thera-peutically useful drugs.

SUMMARY

α-adrenoreceptor antagonists block the actions of noradrenaline and other sympathomimetic substances on postsynaptic α-adrenoreceptors in effector tissues. Most of the drugs of this class produce their actions by competition with α-agonists for α-adrenoreceptors. The earliest reported group of drugs with this action was the ergot alkaloids of which a mixture of the dihydro derivatives of three of the alkaloids (dihydroergotoxine) is used clinically to block α-adrenoreceptors. Other competitive antagonists in clinical use are tolazoline, phentolamine and thymoxamine. Phenoxybenzamine is an α-adrenoreceptor anta-gonist which belongs to a group of compounds, the haloalkyla-mines, which produce a characteristic and persistent non-competitive antagonist effect.

The main clinical uses for α-adrenoreceptor antagonists is in the treatment of conditions characterised by excessive vaso-constriction such as Raynaud's syndrome, in the diagnosis and treatment of phaeochromocytoma and to oppose the vasocon-strictor effects of overdosage with sympathomimetic drugs. As a class the α-adrenoreceptor antagonists are not very specific for α-adrenoreceptors and produce a number of other pharmacological actions. In clinical use the α-adrenoreceptor antagonists produce variable effects on blood pressure and, with the exception of prazosin, are relatively ineffective in the treatment of most forms of hypertension. These drugs usually provoke an increase in cardiac output by causing reflex activation of the sympathetic cardiac nerves resulting from the peripheral vasodilatation which they cause, and also by a presynaptic effect on sympathetic nerves leading to an increased release of transmitter.

Recent work suggests that pre- and postsynaptic α-adrenoreceptors may not be identical and may lead to the production of selective agonists and antagonists of each type of receptor.

REFERENCES

Ahlquist, R. P. (1948) A study of adrenotropic receptors. *Am. J. Physiol.*, **153**, 586–600.

Brown, G. L. & Gillespie, J. S. (1957) The output of sympathetic transmitter from the spleen of the cat. *J. Physiol.*, **138**, 81–102.

Dale, H. H. (1906) On some physiological actions of ergot. *J. Physiol.*, **34**, 163–206.

Nickerson, M. & Goodman, L. S. (1947) Pharmacological properties of a new adrenergic blocking agent: N, N-dibenzyl-β-chloroethylamine (dibenamine). *J. Pharmac. exp. Ther.*, **89**, 167–185.

Starke, K. (1977) Regulation of noradrenaline release by presynaptic receptor systems. *Rev. Physiol. Biochem. Pharmacol.*, **77**, 1–124.

GENERAL READING

Bowman, W. C., Rand, M. J. & West, G. B. (1968) *Textbook of Pharmacology*, Oxford: Blackwell Scientific Publications.

Myers, K. A. (1967) Medical therapy in arterial disorders of the extremities: Vasodilator Drugs. *Modern Treatment*, **4**, 370–385.

Nickerson, M. & Collier, B. (1975) Drugs inhibiting adrenergic nerves and structures innervated by them. *The Pharmacological Basis of Therapeutics*, 5th edn., pp. 533–564, ed. Goodman, L. S. & Gilman, A. New York: Macmillan Publishing Co.

Rose, S. S. (1967) The use and abuse of vasodilator drugs. *Vascular Diseases*, **4**, 67–82.

β-Adrenoreceptor blocking agents

The introduction of substances which selectively blocked β-adrenoreceptors provided the final confirmation of Ahlquist's general classification of adrenoreceptors into α and β types. After 1958 when the first β-adrenoreceptor blocking drug, dichloroisoprenaline, was described it became possible to selectively stimulate or block both α and β-adrenoreceptors which greatly facilitated the analysis of physiological and pharmacological events occurring within the autonomic nervous system. The subsequent recognition and use of β-adrenoreceptor blockers in human therapy contrasts sharply with the historical background of the α-adrenoreceptor blockers described in the previous chapter. From a theoretical standpoint it was predicted that α-adrenoreceptor antagonists might be of value in the treatment of important cardiovascular diseases such as hypertension whereas little therapeutic use could be deduced from the blockade of β-adrenoreceptors. In practice precisely the reverse has been shown to be true. The α-adrenoreceptor antagonists have, in general, been somewhat disappointing therapeutically with few clear-cut indications, whilst the β-adrenoreceptor antagonists have proved to be of great value in the treatment of common and serious conditions such as hypertension, angina pectoris and cardiac arrhythmias.

THE PROTOTYPE β-ADRENORECEPTOR ANTAGONISTS; DICHLOROISOPRENALINE AND PRONETHALOL

The first β-adrenoreceptor antagonist dichloroisoprenaline (usually called DCI) was described by Powell & Slater (1958). It is derived from the β-adrenoreceptor agonist isoprenaline by substitution of chlorine atoms for the hydroxyl groups on the benzene ring (see Fig. 12.1). DCI is a partial agonist, that is it initially stimulates β-adrenoreceptors before blocking them.

Almost all the later β-adrenoreceptor antagonists have the isoprenaline side-chain as part of their molecules and a number of them also have some initial stimulant effects on β-adreno-receptors and this property has been commonly referred to as intrinsic sympathomimetic activity. Powell & Slater (1958) showed that DCI blocked a number of the inhibitory effects of adrenaline in both isolated tissues and in whole animal prepar-ations. This was followed by the important observation of Moran & Perkins (1958) that DCI selectively blocked the cardiac stimulant effects of isoprenaline, adrenaline and sympathetic

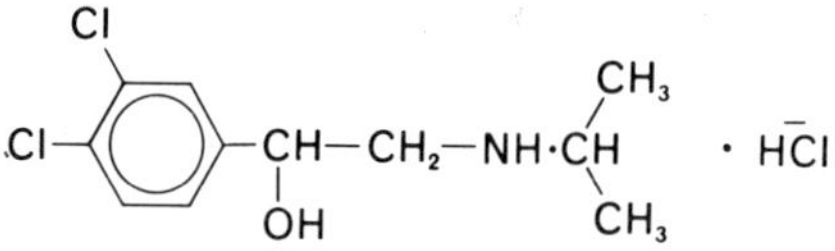

dichloroisoprenaline hydrochloride (DCI)

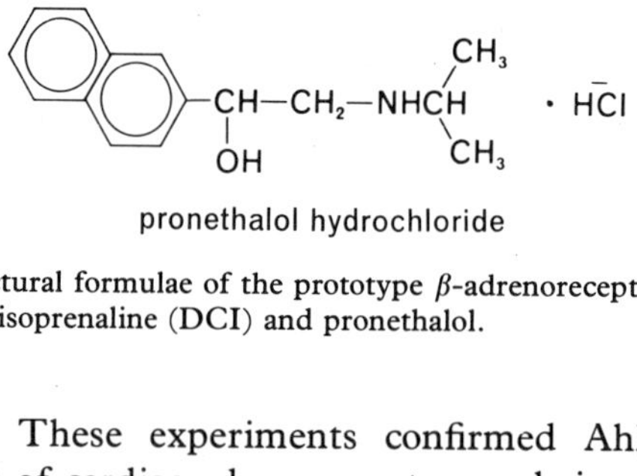

pronethalol hydrochloride

Fig. 12.1 Structural formulae of the prototype β-adrenoreceptor blocking agents dichloroisoprenaline (DCI) and pronethalol.

stimulation. These experiments confirmed Ahlquist's (1948) classification of cardiac adrenoreceptors as being predominantly of the β-type and also provided the starting point for a large number of experimental and clinical studies into the effects of blocking cardiac β-adrenoreceptors. Little consideration was apparently given by the early workers to the possible clinical implications of β-adrenoreceptor blockade. Powell & Slater (1958) wrote 'DCI should prove useful as a tool in the study of pharmacological problems related to adrenergic mechanisms.' DCI was tested in man but its powerful initial β-stimulant effects precluded its detailed examination.

The clinical potentialities of β-adrenoreceptor blocking drugs were first recognised by J. W. Black and his colleagues who noted that in patients suffering from angina pectoris, attacks of anginal pain are often induced by stress such as emotion or exercise which provoke increased sympathetic activity to the heart with a consequent increase in cardiac work and oxygen demand. They reasoned that if the cardiac stimulant effects of sympathetic activation could be prevented by blocking β-adrenoreceptors then the pain of angina might be relieved. Black and his group prepared and tested a number of compounds and the first to show real advantages over DCI was pronethalol (Black & Stephenson, 1962). Pronethalol (Fig. 12.1) is structurally related to both isoprenaline and DCI but in animals and man has much weaker initial stimulant effects than either. In man pronethalol was shown to be effective in the treatment of angina pectoris and also to lower blood pressure in hypertensive patients. Studies of its actions in man were curtailed because of reports that it produced tumours of the thymus glands of mice. However, Black and his colleagues had by this time prepared a non-carcinogenic β-adrenoreceptor blocker more potent than pronethalol and virtually devoid of intrinsic sympathomimetic activity. This substance was called propranolol and was first described by Black, Duncan & Shanks (1965). Propranolol has been widely tested both experimentally and clinically over a number of years and may be considered as the classical agent of this type.

Propranolol hydrochloride BP

$$\text{OCH}_2-\underset{\underset{\text{OH}}{|}}{\text{CH}}-\text{CH}_2-\text{NHCH}\overset{\overset{\text{CH}_3}{/}}{\underset{\underset{\text{CH}_3}{\backslash}}{}} \cdot \text{H}\bar{\text{C}}\text{l}$$

General properties. Propranolol is a potent competitive antagonist of β-adrenoreceptors and is virtually devoid of intrinsic sympathomimetic effect. It is non-selective in its antagonism of β-adrenoreceptors and is equally effective on β_1 and β_2-adrenoreceptors (see Fig. 12.2). Propranolol possesses considerable local anaesthetic activity and is optically active. The isomers of propranolol are equi-active in stabilising cell membranes (i.e. local anaesthetic action) but the ($-$)-isomer is some 50 to 100 times more potent in blocking β-adrenoreceptors than the ($+$)-isomer. The commercially used form of the drug is the racemic mixture. Propranolol is relatively specific in its actions on β-adrenoreceptors and few of its pharmacological actions in animals or man can be ascribed to any other property of the drug. It appears from studies in animals and man that propranolol is only slightly less effective in blocking the effects of sympathetic stimulation to the heart than it is in blocking the effects of exogenously administered β-adrenoreceptor stimulants. In this respect the β-adrenoreceptor antagonists differ from the α-adrenoreceptor antagonists which in tissues containing α-adrenoreceptors are generally much more effective against exogenously administered α-adrenoreceptor stimulants than against the effects of sympathetic nerve stimulation.

Propranolol is well absorbed after oral administration in man but considerable variations in the dose necessary to produce β-adrenoreceptor blockade have been reported between different

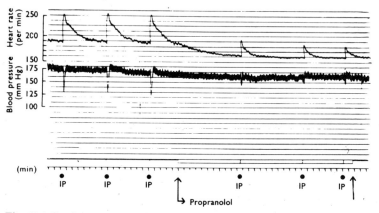

Fig. 12.2 Continuous recordings of arterial blood pressure and heart rate from a chloralose-anaesthetised cat. Intravenous injections of 0.2 micrograms/Kg of isoprenaline (IP) initially caused falls in blood pressure (due to vasodilatation of peripheral blood vessels caused by stimulation of β_2-adrenoreceptors) and increases in heart rate (stimulation of cardiac β_1-adrenoreceptors). The intravenous infusion of propranolol (2.5 micrograms/Kg/min between the arrows) markedly reduced both effects of isoprenaline. (From, Black, Duncan & Shanks, 1965).

individuals. This is probably accounted for by marked inter-patient differences in the rate and extent of metabolism of the drug rather than to changes in absorption. Propranolol is rapidly metabolised by the liver and after an oral dose as much as 50–70 per cent of the absorbed drug may be lost on passage from the intestine to the liver and will not therefore reach the systemic circulation. Clearly differences in the extent of this so-called 'first-pass' effect between patients will have marked effects on the plasma levels of the drug reached in the systemic circulation. Propranolol is a lipid-soluble substance and is widely distributed in the tissues of the body including the central nervous system.

The most important pharmacological actions of propranolol from a clinical standpoint are those exerted on the cardio-vascular and respiratory systems.

Effects on the cardiovascular system. The most significant cardiovascular effects of propranolol are due to blockade of cardiac β-adrenoreceptors. In usual clinical doses propranolol causes bradycardia by blocking the cardiac sympathetic influence and it also reduces the force of cardiac contraction; both effects contribute to the fall in cardiac output which it produces. After acute dosage or in the early stages of chronic administration propranolol increases total peripheral resistance, an effect due partly to blockade of β_2-adrenoreceptors subserving vaso-dilatation and possibly also to compensatory sympathetic reflexes resulting from the reduced cardiac output. Blood flow to all tissues apart from the brain is reduced by propranolol. In normotensive persons propranolol may cause a small fall in blood pressure but in most hypertensive patients it produces a slowly-developing but usually marked lowering of both systolic and diastolic blood pressures. The extent of the lag period between instituting treatment with propranolol and the maximal fall in blood pressure has been the subject of controversy. Some workers have suggested that the full effect may take a week or longer to manifest itself whilst other reports suggest a shorter period of perhaps one or two days. It is likely that part at least of the differences may be accountable for in terms of differences in bio-availability of the drug between different individuals. Another factor may be the extent and duration of the increase in peripheral resistance produced by the drug since this may be sufficient to cancel the effect of the reduced cardiac output and thus leave the blood pressure unaltered. Tarazi & Dustan (1972) showed that in hypertensive patients receiving propranolol there was little fall in blood pressure until the initially increased peripheral resistance returned to (or below) control values. Similarly, in patients who did not respond to propranolol it was found that their peripheral resistance remained elevated. In accordance with this theory is the fact that the β-adrenoreceptor antagonists which are selective for cardiac β-adrenoreceptors and therefore have little effect on peripheral resistance produce a hypotensive effect of more rapid onset.

Propranolol is effective in the prophylactic treatment of angina pectoris and reduces both the number and severity of attacks. In patients suffering from angina the amount of exercise which can be tolerated without anginal pain is increased by cardiac β-adrenoreceptor blockade. The mechanism for this action is complex but depends partly on the reduction in cardiac rate and blood pressure which together reduce the myocardial work load and hence oxygen demand. There is also evidence which suggests that following β-adrenoreceptor blockade the myocardium is able to extract a larger proportion of the oxygen from the blood perfusing it. In normal persons prevention by β-adrenoreceptor blockade of the increase in cardiac output in response to exercise leads to a reduction in the amount of exercise which can be performed.

Propranolol is effective in the treatment of a number of cardiac arrhythmias of both supraventricular and ventricular origin. It was originally thought that this effect, and also the action of propranolol in sometimes precipitating cardiac failure in patients with poor cardiac reserve, were related to the membrane stabilising effects of the drug. However, later studies have shown that both actions are due to β-adrenoreceptor blockade since they are shared by other β-adrenoreceptor antagonists which lack membrane stabilising effects.

Effects on the respiratory system. Smooth muscle in the respiratory tract is relaxed by sympathetic nerve stimulation via an action on β_2-adrenoreceptors and this action is blocked by propranolol leading to an increase in airways resistance. In normal persons this bronchoconstrictor effect is small and of no clinical significance. However, in persons suffering from obstructive airways disease such as asthma or bronchitis then the effect may be very important and may lead to severe bronchoconstriction and respiratory distress. Fatalities have occurred from this cause in asthmatic patients receiving propranolol and it was this potential side-effect which led to the search for, and ultimate introduction of, β-adrenoreceptor blockers having a selective action on the myocardial β_1-adrenoreceptors and which therefore have little effect on the respiratory system (see later).

Effects on the central nervous system. Propranolol readily penetrates into the brain and there is little doubt that it can produce central effects in man. However, it is not clear to what extent antagonism of central β-adrenoreceptors contributes to these central effects. In normal therapeutic doses propranolol produces little obvious effect on mood or on other central functions although vivid dreaming is fairly common and with high doses there have been occasional cases of mental depression and hallucinations. Propranolol has been reported to be of value in the treatment of anxiety states but the site of this action is not clear.

Effects on metabolism. The stimulant effects of sympathetic activity and of sympathomimetics on carbohydrate and fat metabolism are believed to be mediated via β-adrenoreceptors activating the enzyme adenyl cyclase which in turn leads to increased production of cyclic AMP. The precise nature of the β-adrenoreceptors mediating metabolic effects is not clear although the experimental evidence suggests that they more closely resemble β_2 than β_1-adrenoreceptors. In man, propranolol inhibits the rise in plasma free fatty acids induced by sympathetic stimulation or by sympathomimetics. The effects on carbohydrate metabolism are less clear; propranolol prevents the hyperglycaemic response to adrenaline and also the secretion of insulin in response to β-adrenoreceptor stimulants. However, in normal persons it produces little effect on either plasma insulin or glucose levels. Glycogenolysis in heart, skeletal muscle and liver are all to some extent inhibited after β-adrenoreceptor blockade.

Release of the proteolytic enzyme renin from the juxtaglomerular cells of the kidney in response to sympathetic nerve stimulation is mediated via β-adrenoreceptors. Renin release induced by either sympathetic stimulation or by β-adrenoreceptor stimulants is inhibited by propranolol and to a varying degree by other β-adrenoreceptor antagonists and it has been suggested that this effect may be related to the antihypertensive effects of these drugs. However, there are other stimuli, not involving neural pathways, which can induce renin release from the kidney and the role of suppression of renin release in the antihypertensive action of propranolol is controversial and will be discussed more fully later in this chapter.

Clinical uses and doses of propranolol

Angina pectoris. The optimal dose of propranolol in this condition varies widely between patients. The maximum danger of precipitating cardiac failure with propranolol occurs in the early stages of β-adrenoreceptor blockade when sympathetic nervous influence to the heart is first removed. For this reason it is usual to start with small oral doses such as 10 or 20 mg three times daily and to gradually increase this until the desired effect is achieved. Prichard (1976) who has much experience in treating this condition with propranolol has reported that average daily doses of 750 mg were required to treat severe angina in his patients although effective daily doses for individual patients ranged from 60 to 2000 mg. In addition to relieving the number and severity of anginal attacks there is evidence to suggest that propranolol may also reduce the incidence of myocardial infarction in patients suffering from angina.

Cardiac arrhythmias. Propranolol is effective against a number of arrhythmias both of supraventricular and ventricular origin. It is particularly effective against catecholamine-induced arrhythmias such as may occur in surgical stress, thyrotoxicosis and phaeochromocytoma. In the treatment of phaeochromocytoma it is important that an α-adrenoreceptor blocker be given before propranolol since the effect of blockade of β_2-adrenoreceptors in blood vessels in the presence of high levels of circulating catecholamines may cause further vasoconstriction and increase in blood pressure. The usual adult dose in the treatment of cardiac arrhythmias is 10 to 40 mg repeated 3 or 4 times daily. In the emergency treatment of arrhythmias the drug may be given by slow intravenous injection in total doses not usually exceeding 10 mg. When used in this way it is safer to atropinise the patient first (dose 1 to 3 mg) in order to avoid excessive bradycardia.

Propranolol has been used to treat cardiac arrhythmias resulting from overdosage with digitalis. The mechanism of this action is not clear.

Hypertension. Propranolol and some of the other drugs of this class have in recent years established themselves as important drugs in the treatment of hypertension. Their main advantage over many other antihypertensive drugs is their relative freedom from unpleasant side-effects such as postural hypotension and gastrointestinal disturbances. The doses necessary to control hypertension are similar to those required to treat angina and show similarly wide inter-patient variation. The usual commencing dose is 40 mg, repeated 2 or 3 times daily which may be increased by an equal amount at weekly intervals until an adequate response is obtained. Recent evidence suggests that once an adequate antihypertensive effect has been obtained it may be possible to administer propranolol once per day without any marked blood pressure fluctuations. It is known that patient compliance with antihypertensive therapy is related to the number of daily doses which have to be taken and is much higher on once per day schedules. It has been variously estimated that 50–80 per cent of hypertensive patients show a satisfactory blood pressure lowering response to propranolol alone and that this proportion may be further increased by giving propranolol together with another antihypertensive agent such as a thiazide diuretic or a vasodilator such as hydrallazine. The precise mechanism of the antihypertensive effect of propranolol is controversial and will be discussed later.

Other cardiac conditions. Propranolol has been found useful in the treatment of conditions associated with thickening of the walls of the ventricles such that the resistance to ventricular emptying is greatly increased (*hypertrophic obstructive cardio-myopathies*). Propranolol by slowing the heart rate and force of contraction facilitates cardiac outflow and produces a consider-able improvement in cardiac performance particularly during exercise.

The role of β-adrenoreceptor blockers in the treatment of myocardial infarction has not yet been fully evaluated. In addition to reducing the incidence of cardiac arrhythmias following infarction there is also evidence to suggest that propranolol may reduce the extent of the acute damage to the cardiac muscle and also aid in its subsequent recovery. Against these potential advantages in the use of β-adrenoreceptor antagonists must be set the possible dangers of producing further depression of the myocardium in patients who, in general, have a low cardiac reserve.

Anxiety states. There is a growing body of evidence to suggest that propranolol may be effective in the treatment of anxiety states. However it is not yet clear whether this action is mainly central or whether peripheral actions of the drug are also important since propranolol blockade of symptoms such as palpitations, tachycardia and muscle tremor may block an anxiety cycle which is self-sustaining. For instance, propranolol is sometimes dramatically effective in treating acute thyro-toxicosis (thyroid 'storm') which it does by blocking the autono-mic manifestations of the condition without affecting the basic course of the disease. However, it has also been suggested that the anti-anxiety effects of propranolol may be due to an action on the brain perhaps in depressing the outflow of efferent sym-pathetic nerve activity from mid and hindbrain regions to the periphery. Such a mechanism might also at least partly explain the beneficial effects of the drug in angina pectoris and hyper-tension in both of which conditions increased sympathetic nerve activity may play an important role.

Propranolol is officially available (BP, BNF) as tablets each containing 10 mg of the hydrochloride and as an injection con-taining 1 mg in 1 ml ampoules. The same preparations are available, together also with tablets of 40, 80 and 160 mg strength, under the proprietary name of INDERAL.

Side-effects and general precautions in the use of propranolol

Most of the side-effects and precautions in the clinical use of propranolol are ascribable to β-adrenoreceptor blockade. The most obvious drawback to the use of the drug is the danger of precipitating severe cardiac depression in patients with low cardiac reserve or, more rarely, in patients particularly sensitive to β-adrenoreceptor blockade. Propranolol is contra-indicated in patients with 2nd or 3rd degree heart block and the danger of producing excessive cardiac depression can to a large degree be overcome by commencing treatment with low doses and increasing them gradually to achieve a desired therapeutic effect. The drug is contra-indicated in patients suffering from asthma or with a history of bronchospasm. Since propranolol inhibits the metabolic responses to adrenaline it is contra-indicated in diabetic patients or in any patients following prolonged fasting. By virtue of blocking β_2-adrenoreceptors subserving vasodilatation in peripheral blood vessels propranolol may cause symptoms of ischaemia such as cold extremities and may exacerbate these symptoms in patients suffering from Raynaud's syndrome and other peripheral vascular disorders.

There have been several reports of severe anginal attacks and of fatal cardiac arrhythmias occurring in patients in whom propranolol administration has been abruptly withdrawn. These effects appear to be related to the sudden re-institution of sympathetic drive to the myocardium and the risk can be minimised by gradual reduction in the dose of propranolol. Treatment of overdosage with propranolol consists of administering atropine to block vagal influence on the heart and, if necessary, this may be followed by the intravenous administration of a β-adrenoreceptor agonist such as isoprenaline.

Other side-effects of propranolol which cannot be definitely ascribed to β-adrenoreceptor blockade include nausea, insomnia, lassitude, diarrhoea and mental depression. These side-effects usually affect only a minority of patients and can sometimes be overcome by adjustment of dosage.

Other non-selective β-adrenoreceptor antagonists

The gradual recognition of the therapeutic value of propranolol has led to the introduction of a number of other β-adrenoreceptor antagonists into clinical use. These compounds all bear structural similarity to both isoprenaline and propranolol and they differ from each other mainly in potency and in the amount of intrinsic sympathomimetic and/or local anaesthetic potency which they possess. Despite various claims to the contrary there is no convincing evidence that either of these latter properties plays any significant part in the therapeutic efficacy of these drugs. The structures of the non-selective β-adrenoreceptor antagonists at present clinically available are shown in Table 12.1.

Sotalol

The pharmacology of this substance closely resembles that of propranolol. Thus it is of similar β-adrenoreceptor blocking potency, is non-selective in its action on β-adrenoreceptors and is devoid of intrinsic sympathomimetic activity. It differs from propranolol in lacking local anaesthetic action and in being only slowly eliminated, mainly in the unchanged form, from the body. It has been suggested that the local anaesthetic activity of propranolol might relate to both its antiarrhythmic action and also to its effect in precipitating acute cardiac failure in some patients. However, this now seems very unlikely since β-adrenoreceptor blockers such as sotalol without local anaesthetic activity also have antiarrhythmic actions and may induce acute cardiac failure. After single doses of sotalol in man its β-adrenoreceptor blocking action persists longer than that of propranolol and it is often administered only once daily. However it is likely that during chronic therapy with adequate doses then the effective plasma half life of propranolol and probably also of other β-adrenoreceptor blockers may be increased and these too may be effective on a similar dosage schedule.

Clinical uses and dosage. The indications for sotalol, and indeed for all the available β-adrenoreceptor blockers, are the same as those for propranolol. In the treatment of angina pectoris and hypertension the usual starting dose of sotalol is 80 mg given twice daily for the first 7 to 10 days and then increased if necessary to 200 to 600 mg per day given either as a single dose or in divided doses. In the treatment of cardiac arrhythmias and thyrotoxicosis the usual oral daily dose is 120 to 240 mg. The drug is commercially available under the proprietary name of BETA-CARDONE as tablets each containing 40, 80 or 200 mg of the hydrochloride and as an injection containing 10 mg in 5 ml. It is also available as 80 mg strength tablets under the proprietary name of SOTACOR.

Alprenolol hydrochloride BP

This substance has more marked intrinsic sympathomimetic

Table 12.1 *Non-selective β-adrenoreceptor blockers*

structure	approved name	proprietary name(s)
	sotalol hydrochloride	BETA-CARDONE SOTACOR
	alprenolol hydrochloride B.P.	—
	oxprenolol hydrochloride	TRASICOR
	pindolol	VISKEN
	timolol maleate	BLOCADREN

activity than propranolol but otherwise has similar pharmacological actions and therapeutic uses.

Clinical use and dosage. In the treatment of angina and hypertension the usual starting dose is 50 mg given 4 times daily which may be gradually increased up to 100 mg four times daily. Cardiac arrhythmias usually respond to doses between 25 and 50 mg given 3 or 4 times daily but up to a total dose of 400 mg per day may be necessary in some individuals. The drug may be used intravenously in usual doses of 2 to 5 mg in the treatment of cardiac arrhythmias. The official (BP) preparations are tablets of 50 mg and an injection containing 1 mg in 1 ml.

Oxprenolol

This substance has more intrinsic sympathomimetic activity and less local anaesthetic potency than propranolol but is of similar potency in antagonising the effects of β-adrenoreceptor stimulation. It has been reported that the maximal reduction in heart rate obtainable in patients receiving β-adrenoreceptor antagonists such as oxprenolol and pindolol, having marked sympathomimetic effects, is less than that achieved with substances such as propranolol having little or no intrinsic stimulant activity. This observation has been extrapolated to the suggestion that drugs having intrinsic sympathomimetic activity may have a reduced tendency to precipitate cardiac failure. There is not, however, any convincing evidence to support this suggestion.

Clinical uses and dosage. In the treatment of angina and hypertension the usual starting doses of oxprenolol are in the range of 40 to 80 mg given two or three times daily. Most patients respond to daily doses between 120 and 480 mg although occasionally patients may require 960 mg. Cardiac arrhythmias often respond to doses of 20 to 40 mg given three times daily but the dose may need to be increased in some patients. In the emergency treatment of cardiac arrhythmias the drug may be given either intramuscularly or intravenously in doses of 1 to 2 mg which may be repeated, if necessary, after 10 to 20 minutes. When given parenterally the drug is often preceded by the intravenous administration of 1 to 2 mg of atropine sulphate to prevent excessive bradycardia. Oxprenolol is officially (BNF) available as tablets of 20 mg strength and also under the proprietary name of TRASICOR as tablets of 20, 40, 80 and 160 mg strength and as ampoules each containing 2 mg of the hydrochloride as solid intended for making up injections. A slow-release tablet formulation containing 160 mg of the hydrochloride (SLOW-TRASICOR) has recently been introduced and is intended for the once-daily treatment of hypertension.

Pindolol

This substance differs from the other non-selective β-adreno-receptor blockers in having the highest potency in terms of both β-adrenoreceptor antagonism and intrinsic sympathomimetic activity of the clinically available compounds of this class.

Clinical uses and dosage. In the treatment of hypertension the initial daily dosage is 5 to 15 mg which may be gradually increased to 45 mg. Recent studies have shown that the drug produces a smooth control of high blood pressure when the total daily dose is given on a single occasion thus greatly improving patient compliance with therapy. It has been reported that in hypertensive patients treated with pindolol approximately 5 per cent of patients may respond with an increase in blood pressure instead of a lowering and that in the majority of these the hypotensive effect of pindolol may be revealed if the dose is lowered to approximately half the previous level. The reason for this curious effect is not known. The effective doses of pindolol in the treatment of angina pectoris are usually somewhat less than those used in hypertension. The drug is not recommended for the treatment of cardiac arrhythmias presumably on account of its potent initial cardiac stimulant properties.

Pindolol is commercially available as 5 mg tablets under the proprietary name of VISKEN.

Timolol

This substance has high potency in blocking β-adrenoreceptors but has little local anaesthetic or intrinsic sympathomimetic activity.

Clinical uses and dosage. In the treatment of hypertension and angina it is usual to commence treatment with daily doses of 10 to 15 mg which may then be gradually increased, at intervals of not less than three days, to produce the desired response. Most hypertensive patients respond to total daily dosage of 30 mg but this may sometimes be increased to a recommended total dose of 60 mg. In the treatment of angina the majority of patients respond to a daily dose of 35 to 45 mg. Timolol is usually administered in divided doses two or three times daily although it may well be that it too would be effective on a once a day regimen.

Timolol is not at present recommended for the treatment of cardiac arrhythmias.

The drug is available as tablets each containing 10 mg of the maleate under the proprietary name of BLOCADREN.

Antagonists selective for β_1-adrenoreceptors

A major disadvantage in the clinical use of non-selective β-adrenoreceptor antagonists such as propranolol is that they increase airways resistance, an effect which may precipitate bouts of acute bronchospasm in patients suffering from asthma or other obstructive airways conditions. The mechanism of this bronchospasm is not entirely clear but is probably related to unopposed parasympathetic activity in persons predisposed to bronchoconstriction. The confirmation by many workers of the sub-classification of β-adrenoreceptors into β_1 and β_2-types opened the theoretical possibility of producing antagonists with a selective action on the β_1-adrenoreceptors of the myocardium. The first cardioselective compound to be extensively used in man was practolol which was introduced into clinical use in 1970. This drug has since been withdrawn from general clinical use because of toxic effects apparently unrelated to β-adreno-receptor blockade. It remains, however, the prototype drug of the cardioselective agents. It is important to remember that these substances are cardioselective rather than cardiospecific and in sufficient dosage they have been shown to block β_2-adrenoreceptors in the respiratory tract and elsewhere.

Practolol

$$CH_3CONH-\!\!\left\langle\bigcirc\right\rangle\!\!-OCH_2-\underset{\underset{OH}{|}}{CH}-CH_2-NHCH\underset{CH_3}{\overset{CH_3}{<}}$$

Practolol differs from propranolol in a number of respects; it is a water-soluble compound, is practically devoid of local anaes-thetic activity and possesses moderate intrinsic sympathomimetic activity. However, the most important difference from proprano-lol is that it has a more marked blocking action on the β_1-adrenoreceptors of the heart than on the β_2-adrenoreceptors of the respiratory tract. Vaughan Williams, Bagwell & Singh (1973) showed in dogs that practolol was eight times more active in blocking cardiac (β_1) than peripheral vascular (β_2) adreno-receptors. These workers also showed that the cardioselectivity of practolol was associated with the position of the substituent group on the benzene ring. If the group was moved from the para to the ortho position then cardioselectivity was lost. Practolol, unlike propranolol, is only metabolised by liver enzymes to a small extent and some 80–90 per cent of an oral dose of the drug is excreted unchanged in the urine. The high water-solubility of practolol compared to that of propranolol results in somewhat different distributions of the two compounds in the body fluids. Thus practolol penetrates into the brain at a slow rate and reaches a much lower concentration than do lipid soluble substances such as propranolol. The low degree of penetration into the central nervous system of practolol has been construed by some workers to be evidence against it having important central effects. However the evidence is by no means conclusive since it is known that much of the propranolol which is detectable in brain tissue is in the form of metabolites whereas it is likely that a high proportion of the practolol would be in the unchanged and presumably more active form. Some workers have also suggested that practolol has a reduced tendency over propranolol to induce cardiac failure. This suggestion has not yet been confirmed either in the case of practolol or using other cardioselective agents.

Clinical uses and dosage. Practolol is effective in all conditions for which propranolol has been used. The usual daily doses in the treatment of hypertension and angina are in the range 200 to 300 mg although doses up to 1·2 g have been used. It may also be used orally or intravenously to treat disturbances of cardiac rhythm. The intravenous dose range is usually 5 to 20 mg. In patients suffering from obstructive airways conditions such as bronchial asthma practolol may be used concurrently with a sympathomimetic substance such as isoprenaline or salbutamol.

Toxicity

From its introduction in 1970 the incidence of reported toxic reactions to practolol was much higher than for other β-adreno-receptor blockers; the most common reaction being a psoriasis-like skin rash which slowly cleared on discontinuing the drug. However, in some patients there is a reaction in the eyes leading to a reduction in tear production, scarring of the conjunctiva and occasionally to blindness ('dry red eyes syndrome'). It has been estimated that there have been about 500 eye reactions in the United Kingdom though not all have led to blindness. Another serious toxic reaction to practolol, which has thus far been positively identified in less than 100 cases, is sclerosing peritonitis. In this condition, which has probably led to loss of life, layers of peritoneum and intestine may become fused together forming severe intestinal adhesions. The precise mechanisms for these toxic effects of practolol have not been determined but they appear to be unrelated to β-adrenoreceptor blockade since they are not shown by other antagonists either of the non-selective or cardioselective groups. Practolol was withdrawn from general clinical use in 1975 and it is now restricted to hospital use only, where it is mainly used to treat cardiac arrhythmias. For this use it is available as tablets of 100 mg strength and as an injection containing 2 mg/ml in 5 ml ampoules; the proprietary name is ERALDIN.

With the introduction of less toxic cardioselective substances (Table 12.2) there seems little justification for the continued clinical use of practolol.

Metoprolol

This substance is of similar potency to propranolol in blocking cardiac β_1-adrenoreceptors but is much less active in blocking the β_2-adrenoreceptors of the respiratory tract and peripheral vasculature. It resembles propranolol in being extensively metabolised in the body, in having local anaesthetic potency and in being practically devoid of intrinsic sympathomimetic activity.

Clinical uses and dosage. To treat hypertension metoprolol is administered in starting doses of 100 mg given twice daily and this may be subsequently increased if necessary to 200 mg twice daily. Some recent reports have shown that the drug provides satsfactory control of blood pressure when given only once per day. In the treatment of angina pectoris most patients respond to doses of 50 to 100 mg repeated twice or three times daily. Metoprolol is available as tablets of 50 and 100 mg strength (proprietary names LOPRESSOR and BETALOC).

Acebutolol

This substance has both local anaesthetic and intrinsic sympathomimetic activity; in most respects it is similar in its actions to other drugs in this sub-group.

Clinical use and dosage. Acebutolol is recommended for the treatment of angina, hypertension and cardiac arrhythmias. Angina patients usually respond to 400 mg daily given in divided doses but some patients may require more with a practical

Table 12.2   *Antagonists selective for β_1-adrenoreceptors*

structure	approved name	proprietary name(s)
$CH_3OCH_2CH_2$—⟨phenyl⟩—$OCH_2 \cdot CH - CH_2 - NHCH(CH_3)_2$, OH · tartrate	metoprolol tartrate	BETALOC LOPRESSOR
$CH_3CH_2CH_2CONH$—⟨phenyl, $COCH_3$⟩—$OCH_2 - CH - CH_2 \cdot NHCH(CH_3)_2$, OH · $\overline{H}Cl$	acebutolol hydrochloride	SECTRAL
$H_2N \cdot CO \cdot CH_2$—⟨phenyl⟩—$OCH_2 - CH - CH_2NHCH(CH_3)_2$, OH	atenolol	TENORMIN

maximum of 1·2 g per day. In the treatment of hypertension treatment is usually started with twice daily doses of 200 mg but may be increased if necessary by increments up to 600 mg twice daily. Cardiac arrhythmias may be treated with oral daily doses of 300 to 600 mg or by intravenous doses of 5 to 25 mg.

Acebutolol is commercially available under the proprietary name of SECTRAL as capsules of 100 and 200 mg strength and as an injection of 5 mg per ml strength in 5 ml ampoules.

Atenolol
This cardioselective substance lacks both local anaesthetic and intrinsic sympathomimetic activity. The drug is well absorbed by mouth, is mostly excreted unchanged in the urine and has a biological half-life in man long enough to allow of once a day dosage in the treatment of hypertension.

Clinical use and dosage. Atenolol is recommended for the treatment of hypertension in which it has been shown to be effective in once daily doses of 50 to 200 mg. It appears to be effective alone in about 75 per cent of hypertensive patients and there is apparently little difference in the hypotensive effects obtained with doses over the range of 50 to 200 mg per day. It is available as tablets of 100 mg strength (proprietary name TENORMIN).

Compounds which block both α and β-adrenoreceptors

Labetalol

This compound, which is thus far the only member of this group available for clinical use, has the novel actions of competitively antagonising the effects of stimulating both α and β-adreno-receptors. Its experimental pharmacology was first described by Farmer, Kennedy, Levy & Marshall (1972) who showed that the β-adrenoreceptor blocking component of labetalol's action was non-selective and was more potent than its α-adreno-receptor antagonist effect. In animal experiments it was shown to be 5 to 18 times less potent than propranolol in blocking β-adrenoreceptors and, like propranolol, it has local anaesthetic activity but no significant intrinsic sympathomimetic action. As an α-adrenoreceptor antagonist it was shown to be 2 to 7 times less potent than phentolamine. Labetalol lowers blood pressure in both animals and man, and in animal experiments it has been shown to protect the heart from catecholamine-induced arrhythmias. The rationale for the use of labetalol in the treatment of hypertension is that it will produce vasodilatation of peripheral blood vessels due to its α-adrenoreceptor antagonist action, but the effects of the reflex increase in sympathetic activity to the heart normally caused by this type of action is abolished by the blockade of cardiac β-adrenoreceptors produced. It is claimed that the resultant of these actions should be a reduction in cardiac output together with an increase in peripheral blood flow and therefore a more 'normal' circulation than is the case with substances which block only one type of adrenoreceptor. The drug has thus far had only a limited clinical usage and it is too early to decide whether the theoretical advantages claimed for it will be fully translated into tangible benefit to the hypertensive patient.

Clinical use and dosage. Labetalol is recommended for the treatment of hypertension of all grades of severity. The recommended oral daily dosage is between 300 mg and 2·4 g in divided doses. Symptoms of peripheral sympathetic nerve blockade such as postural hypotension, nasal stuffiness and failure of ejaculation have been reported by some patients. The drug has also been used intravenously in doses of 50 to 200 mg to produce a rapid lowering of blood pressure in hypertensive crises. The drug is commercially available (proprietary name TRANDATE) as tablets of 100 and 200 mg strength and as an injection of 5 mg/ml strength in 20 ml ampoules.

Mechanism of action of β-adrenoreceptor antagonists in the treatment of hypertension

Although it was not predicted that β-adrenoreceptor antagonists would lower arterial blood pressure in man it is this action of these substances which has assumed the most clinical significance. In the last quarter of a century there has been an increasing recognition of the role played by elevated blood pressure in the incidence of cardiovascular disorders such as angina, congestive heart failure, stroke and myocardial infarction. The fact that deaths from cardiovascular disease in Western civilisations outnumber the combined deaths from all other causes led Caldwell (1976) to write, 'High blood pressure is slowing being recognised as the leading preventable cause of death and disability.'

Other effective antihypertensives available include ganglion blockers (Chapter 7), noradrenergic neurone blockers (Chapter 10) and centrally acting substances such as α-methylDOPA and clonidine (Chapter 13). However, the great interest in the β-adrenoreceptor antagonists as antihypertensive agents stems from their lack of side-effects in clinical use. They do not inhibit sympathetic reflexes involved in postural changes or during exercise nor do they interfere with gastrointestinal activity or with sexual function. Clearly, as a group the β-adrenoreceptor antagonists are acceptable to most hypertensive patients and the fact that many of them produce smooth control of blood pressure when taken only once daily makes patient compliance with therapy more likely and may perhaps lead to a fall in the number of preventable deaths from the sequelae of hypertension. Another practical advantage of the β-adreno-receptor blockers is that they are compatible with other anti-hypertensive agents with which they usually produce additive effects.

The precise mechanism by which β-adrenoreceptor antagonists lower blood pressure is not yet clear but has been subjected to intensive investigation and some speculation. The simplest suggested mechanism is that they reduce cardiac output by inhibiting sympathetic excitatory influence whilst producing little effect on peripheral resistance. However, there have been several reports of differences in the time course of cardiac β-adrenoreceptor blockade and the onset of the hypotensive response and also in the dose of the drug necessary to produce the two effects. Despite early suggestions to the contrary it now seems certain that the antihypertensive effect of these drugs is mediated via β-adrenoreceptor blockade and that other actions such as local anaesthesia and intrinsic sympathomimetic action are unlikely to play a significant role. Many clinical workers have reported a delay from commencing treatment with β-adrenoreceptor blocking agents before the onset of the anti-hypertensive effect. This delay is accountable in the case of propranolol, which has been most studied, by differences in metabolism and bioavailability of the drug between patients and, secondly, by the fact that the drug causes an initial increase in peripheral resistance which may offset the fall in cardiac output and result in little change in blood pressure. The problem is complicated by the fact that most patients are started on low doses of the drug and a considerable time may elapse before an effective therapeutic level is reached in the body. The cardio-selective drugs, such as atenolol, do not, in general, cause any marked change in peripheral resistance and the onset of their antihypertensive action is generally quicker than that of prop-ranolol. However it has been reported that these drugs may take up to a week to produce their full therapeutic effect. The delay in the onset of action of these drugs has been interpreted by some workers to suggest that β-adrenoreceptor blockers may have actions on nervous pathways to the cardiovascular system in addition to their known effect in blocking postsynaptic β-adrenoreceptors. Weight is given to this argument by the fact that most drugs in this group have produced central effects in man and effects on the peripheral nervous system in animals. Animal experimentation has yielded data to suggest that both α and β-adrenoreceptors exist in the mammalian brain which may play a role in the control of efferent sympathetic nerve traffic to the cardiovascular system. Stimulation of α-adreno-receptors located in the medulla oblongata leads to a fall in both peripheral sympathetic nerve activity and arterial blood pressure (see Chapter 13) whilst β-adrenoreceptor stimulation may lead to opposing effects with a consequent increase in blood pressure. It is known that substances such as clonidine stimulate central α-adrenoreceptors and thereby lower blood pressure and it has been speculated that β-adrenoreceptor antagonists, by blocking opposing excitatory effects, would also produce hypotensive effects. The evidence for this type of action is inconclusive (see Day & Roach, 1974) since some of the β-adrenoreceptor blockers, such as practolol and atenolol, are highly polar compounds and penetrate into the brain only slowly and to a small extent and yet are effective antihypertensive agents.

It is also possible that β-adrenoreceptor blockers have important effects on peripheral sympathetic nerves via a pre-synaptic action. Propranolol prevents the release of noradrenaline from a number of sympathetic nerves in isolated smooth muscle preparations (see Fig. 12.3 and review by Weinstock, 1977). Since there is recent evidence to suggest that there exist pre-synaptic β-adrenoreceptors on noradrenergic nerves whose function is to promote the release of noradrenaline then it has been speculated that the blocking action of β-adrenoreceptor antagonists may be exerted on these. However, it is also possible that the noradrenergic neurone blocking action of propranolol may be related to the local anaesthetic action of the drug rather than to a specific effect on β-adrenoreceptors. The lack of a peripheral sympathetic nerve blocking action of β-adreno-receptor antagonists in man is also suggested by the absence of symptoms such as postural hypotension and nasal stuffiness.

Much attention has been given in recent years to the possi-bility that β-adrenoreceptor antagonists lower elevated blood

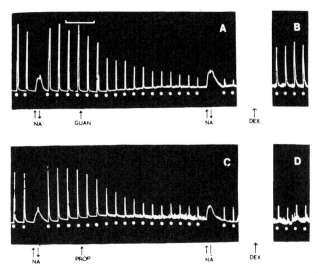

Fig. 12.3 Rat isolated vas deferens preparations. At white dots the sympathetic nerves to the preparations were stimulated for 10 seconds which caused the smooth muscle to contract; the contractions were reduced by the addition to the bath of either 1 microgram/ml of guanethidine (upper record) or 3 micrograms/ml propranolol (lower record). The blocking action of each drug was apparently presynaptic since in neither case were the contractions induced by 2 micrograms/ml noradrenaline reduced. However, the mechanism of the blockade produced by each drug were apparently different since 0·05 microgram/ml of dexamphetamine antagonised the action of guanethidine but not that of propranolol. (From Day, Owen & Warren, 1968).

pressure by suppressing release of renin from the juxtaglo-merular cells of the kidney. In both animals and man renin release may be induced by sympathetic stimulation and by β-adrenoreceptor stimulants such as isoprenaline. The role of renin in the aetiology of hypertension is not known although the angiotensin II which it produces by acting on plasma globulins is a potent vasoconstrictor and releases aldosterone from the cortical cells of the adrenal glands. Aldosterone has a potent effect on the kidney tubules promoting retention of sodium and water with a consequent increase in plasma volume. It seems that human hypertension is multi-factorial and there is no clear correlation between plasma renin levels and the level of blood pressure in most hypertensive patients. However, Bühler, Laragh, Baer, Vaughan & Brunner (1972) showed that patients with high plasma renin levels responded with a more marked fall in blood pressure to β-adrenoreceptor blockers than did patients with normal or low levels. This interesting finding has not been generally confirmed by other workers and differences have been found between the doses necessary to suppress plasma renin levels and those needed to lower blood pressure. Similarly, there are differences in the time course of the suppression of plasma renin and the antihypertensive effects with different antagonists. The problem is somewhat obscured by differences between workers in such factors as selection of patients, assay methods and doses of β-adrenoreceptor antagonists used. It may be that the results of Bühler and his colleagues are most applicable to those patients with high plasma renin in whom the hypertension is apparently largely sustained by the vascular actions of angiotensin II. It appears that such patients may form only a small proportion of the total population of hypertensives.

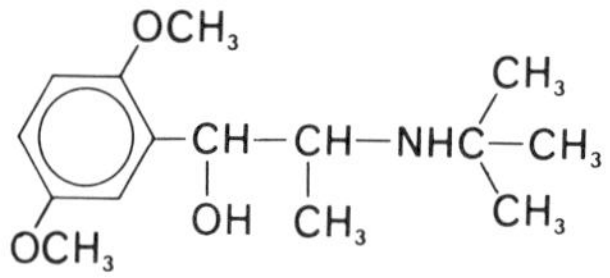

Butoxamine

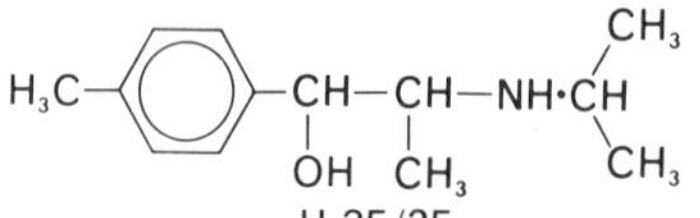

H 35/25

Fig. 12.4 Structural formulae of two compounds which selectively block β_2-adrenoreceptors.

Antagonists selective for β_2-adrenoreceptors: butoxamine and H35/25

These compounds whose structures are shown in Fig. 12.4 have been shown to produce a selective competitive antagonism of the β_2-adrenoreceptors of the respiratory tract, the uterus and those in voluntary muscle involved in tremor. Although of considerable theoretical and experimental interest no clinical uses have yet been proposed for these substances.

SUMMARY

The introduction of substances which produced a selective and competitive antagonism of the effects of β-adrenoreceptor stimulation provided the final piece of experimental evidence to vindicate Ahlquist's classification of adrenoreceptors. The earliest β-adrenoreceptor antagonist, DCI, is structurally closely related to the β-adrenoreceptor stimulant isoprenaline and the subsequently developed β-adrenoreceptor blockers also bear structural similarity to isoprenaline. DCI is a partial agonist, initially stimulating β-adrenoreceptors before blocking them and is as a result unsuitable for widespread clinical use. This intrinsic sympathomimetic effect is virtually absent in propranolol which is the most studied substance in this group of compounds. Propranolol competitively antagonises the effects of stimulating both β_1 and β_2-adrenoreceptors in animals and man and is therefore known as a non-selective β-adrenoreceptor antagonist. The most important pharmacological effects of propranolol are exerted in the cardiovascular system and appear to result from blockade of cardiac β-adrenoreceptors; it causes bradycardia, reduces blood pressure and abolishes the effects of sympathomimetic substances on the heart. In man it is used clinically in the treatment of angina pectoris, hypertension and cardiac arrhythmias. Propranolol is also clinically effective in producing symptomatic improvement in conditions such as anxiety and thyrotoxicosis and further clinical uses are at present under investigation. Inherent dangers in the clinical use of β-adrenoreceptor antagonists such as propranolol are the potential precipitation of heart failure in patients with low cardiac reserve and of bronchoconstriction in patients suffering from asthma or obstructive airways disorders. A number of other non-selective β-adrenoreceptor antagonists are available clinically such as oxprenolol, sotalol and pindolol; these agents differ from propranolol in terms of potency, local anaesthetic effect and/or intrinsic sympathomimetic activity.

Practolol is the prototype of a class of β-adrenoreceptor antagonist which is selective for β_1-adrenoreceptors and in clinical use is less likely to precipitate bronchoconstriction in susceptible patients. Practolol has been withdrawn from general clinical use because of toxicity unrelated to β-adrenoreceptor blockade and has been replaced by less toxic cardioselective agents such as atenolol, metoprolol and acebutolol. The cardioselective β-adrenoreceptor antagonists have the same clinical uses as the non-selective agents.

The antihypertensive action of β-adrenoreceptor antagonists has assumed considerable therapeutic importance because these agents produce an effective lowering of arterial blood pressure without many of the side-effects produced by other antihypertensive drugs. The hypotensive action of β-adrenoreceptor antagonists is mediated mainly by a lowering of cardiac output although the precise mechanism whereby this is brought about is not known. It has been suggested that in addition to blocking postsynaptic β-adrenoreceptors these drugs may have important actions on the sympathetic nervous system at central and/or at peripheral sites. Similarly, some of these drugs have been shown to suppress renin release from the kidney and this action has also been implicated in their antihypertensive effects.

REFERENCES

Ahlquist, R. P. (1948) A study of the adrenotropic receptors. *Am. J. Physiol.*, **153**, 586–600.

Black, J. W. & Stephenson, J. S. (1962) Pharmacology of a new adrenergic beta-receptor blocking compound (Nethalide). *Lancet*, **ii**, 311–314.

Black, J. W., Duncan, W. A. M. & Shanks, R. G. (1965) Comparison of some properties of pronethalol and propranolol. *Br. J. Pharmac.*, **25**, 577–591.

Bühler, F. R., Laragh, J. H., Baer, L., Vaughan, E. D., Jr., & Brunner, H. R. (1972) Propranolol inhibition of renin secretion. A specific approach to diagnosis and treatment of renin-dependent hypertensive diseases. *New Engl. J. Med.*, **287**, 1209–1214.

Caldwell, J. R. (1976) Perspectives in Hypertension—1976. *Geriatrics*, **31**, 46–47.

Day, M. D. & Roach, A. G. (1974) Central adrenoreceptors and the control of arterial blood pressure. *Clin. exp. Pharmac. Physiol.*, **1**, 347–360.

Day, M. D., Owen, D. A. A. & Warren, P. R. (1968) An adrenergic neurone blocking action of propranolol in isolated tissues. *J. Pharm. Pharmac.*, **20**, 130–134s.

Farmer, J. B., Kennedy, I., Levy, G. P. & Marshall, R. J. (1972) Pharmacology of AH5158; a drug which blocks both α and β-adrenoceptors. *Br. J. Pharmac.*, **45**, 660–675.

Moran, N. C. & Perkins, M. E. (1958) Adrenergic blockade of the mammalian heart by a dichloro analogue of isoproterenol. *J. Pharmac. exp. Ther.*, **124**, 233–237.

Powell, C. E. & Slater, I. H. (1958) Blocking of inhibitory adrenergic receptors by a dichloro analog of isoproterenol. *J. Pharmac. exp. Ther.*, **122**, 480–488.

Prichard, B. N. C. (1976) Propranolol in the treatment of angina: a review. *Postgrad. Med. J.*, **52**, Supplement 4, 35–41.

Tarazi, R. C. & Dustan, H. P. (1972) Beta adrenergic blockade in hypertension. Practical and theoretical implications of long-term hemodynamic variations. *Amer. J. Cardiol.*, **29**, 633–640.

Vaughan Williams, E. M., Bagwell, E. E. & Singh, B. N. (1973) Cardiospecificity of β-receptor blockade. A comparison of the relative potencies on cardiac and peripheral vascular β-adrenoceptors of propranolol, of practolol and its ortho-substituted isomer, and of oxprenolol and its para-substituted isomer. *Cardiovasc. Res.*, **7**, 226–240.

Weinstock, M. (1976) The presynaptic effect of β-adrenoceptor antagonists on noradrenergic neurones. *Life Sciences*, **19**, 1453–1466.

GENERAL READING

Chung, E. K. (1974) Beta-blockers in the treatment of disturbances in cardiac rhythm. In Beta-blockers—present status and future prospects, pp 216–229, ed. Schweizèr, E. Berne: Hans Huber Publishers.

Prichard, B. N. C. (1974) β-Adrenergic receptor blocking drugs in angina pectoris. *Drugs*, **7,** 55–84.

Simpson, F. O. (1974) β-Adrenergic receptor blocking drugs in hypertension. *Drugs*, **7,** 85–105.

Shand, D. G. (1975) Propranolol. *New Eng. J. Med.*, **293,** (6) 280–285.

Various authors (1976) Ten years of propranolol, *Postgrad. Med. J.*, **52,** Supplement 4.

Weetman, D. F. (1977) A review of the actions and clinical uses of beta-adrenoceptor blocking drugs. *Medicamentos de Actualidad—Drugs of Today*, **13,** 261–305.

13

Drugs affecting the storage and release of transmitter from noradrenergic neurones

In previous chapters drugs have been described which reduce the release of noradrenaline from sympathetic nerves either by blocking transmission of impulses across sympathetic ganglia (Chapter 7) or by acting on the terminal varicosities of the nerves (Chapter 10). These substances are used clinically to lower arterial blood pressure and their main actions are exerted on peripheral sympathetic nerves. However, some drugs which are used to treat human hypertension affect the storage and/or release of noradrenaline from both central and peripheral noradrenergic neurones and their precise mechanism of action is therefore more difficult to elucidate. Such drugs include the rauwolfia alkaloids, α-methylDOPA, clonidine and monoamine oxidase inhibitors; the actions and clinical uses of these substances will be discussed in the present chapter.

RESERPINE AND OTHER ALKALOIDS FROM RAUWOLFIA

Rauwolfia is a flowering shrub indigenous to India and surrounding countries; a number of varieties exist of which *rauwolfia serpentina* is the most widely used. Approximately 50 different alkaloids have been isolated from the plant of which reserpine is the most important clinically. The highest concentrations of alkaloids are present in the roots but various extracts and preparations of the plant have for centuries been used in Indian folk-medicine to treat conditions ranging from snake bite to insanity. Rauwolfia alkaloids were only introduced into Western medicine in the 1950's following the isolation of reserpine in 1952. The chemical structures of the more important reserpine-like alkaloids are shown in Fig. 13.1.

Reserpine BP

The most striking pharmacological effects of reserpine after administration to either animals or man are those exerted on the brain and gastrointestinal tract. In laboratory animals, such as rats or cats, reserpine produces a characteristic syndrome of effects in which the animal remains motionless in a huddled posture for long periods. The condition is often accompanied by pilo-erection, shivering and diarrhoea. Despite their apparently sedated state reserpinised animals are easily aroused by sensory stimulation and this type of behavioural pattern has been called tranquillisation to distinguish it from the effects produced by frankly sedative substances such as the barbiturates which generally increase the threshold for arousal.

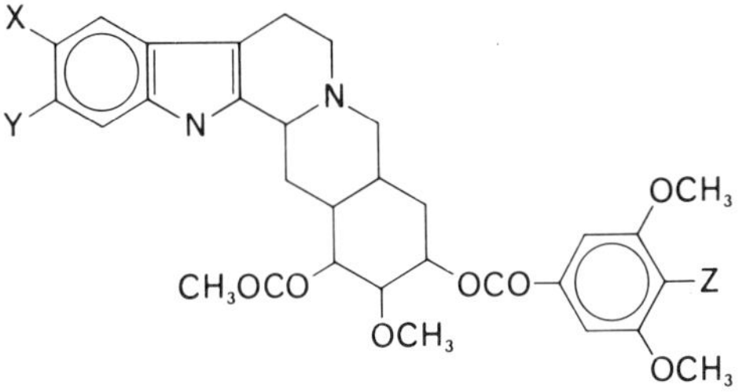

	X	Y	Z
Reserpine	H	OCH₃	—OCH₃
Deserpidine	H	H	—OCH₃
Methoserpidine	OCH₃	H	—OCH₃
Syrosingopine	OCH₃	H	—OCOCH₂CH₃

Fig. 13.1 Structural formulae of reserpine and related substances.

These effects of reserpine are a consequence of its action in disrupting the storage mechanisms for biogenic amines and related substances in nervous tissue both in the brain and in peripheral tissues. Reserpine treatment profoundly lowers the amounts of the catecholamines dopamine, noradrenaline and adrenaline present in tissues and also of other suggested transmitter substances including 5-HT, ATP and γ-aminobutyric acid (GABA). It is not yet clear which of the pharmacological actions of reserpine are of most significance to its clinical uses. It has been variously postulated by different groups of workers that loss of neuronal 5-HT and/or catecholamines are responsible for the tranquillising action of the drug. It seems likely that the peripheral effects of the drug are mainly mediated via depletion of catecholamines, most importantly noradrenaline, from noradrenergic nerves. This peripheral depletion causes an impairment of responses to sympathetic stimulation including the constrictor fibres to blood vessels which results therefore in vasodilatation and a fall in arterial blood pressure. The intestinal over-activity caused by reserpine is probably largely due to the imbalance caused in the autonomic control of the intestine consequent upon the reduction in sympathetic inhibitory influence and resulting therefore in a predominance of para-sympathetic activity. In this respect the action of reserpine resembles that of the noradrenergic neurone blocking agents (Chapter 10). It is likely that the diarrhoea caused by reserpine is also partly due to liberation of 5-HT from enterochromaffin cells of the gut which then exerts direct stimulant effects on the intestinal smooth muscle.

Reserpine was at one time widely used clinically both as a tranquilliser and as an antihypertensive agent. Its use in the treatment of mental illness has greatly declined in recent years because in general it is less effective and produces more unwanted effects than do other available agents such as the phenothiazine derivatives. A major drawback in the clinical use of reserpine is its tendency to cause lethargy and severe mental depression sometimes resulting in suicidal tendencies. In many ways the depression of mood produced by reserpine in both animals and man closely resembles the clinical condition of endogenous depression and reserpine-treated animals therefore form a convenient experimental model of human depressive illness. When used to treat hypertension reserpine is effective in lower doses than are used to treat mental illness and this fact, together with its concurrent use with other antihypertensive agents, does much to reduce the incidence of unwanted actions and to im-prove its clinical effectiveness.

The mechanism of the catecholamine-depleting action of reserpine in noradrenergic nerves
Reserpine causes a marked lowering of the noradrenaline content of most tissues in both animals and man. This effect of reserpine is dose-dependent but the depletion is relatively slow and in many studies large doses have been used for short periods whereas similar degrees of noradrenaline depletion are ob-tainable with much lower doses given over longer periods. The depleting action of reserpine has been most studied in rats and in this species a single dose of about 0.1 mg/kg produces a depletion of cardiac noradrenaline stores which is detectable after about an hour and virtually complete by 12 to 24 hours. The tissue

noradrenaline levels then remain very low for several days and recovery to control levels may take 7 to 14 days. All tissues are not equally susceptible to the action of reserpine; the heart in most species is readily depleted whilst the adrenal medullae are relatively resistant. Only occasionally do sympathomimetic symptoms accompany reserpine administration and this suggests that the mechanism of the depletion is not direct displacement of neuronal noradrenaline by reserpine as occurs, for instance, with indirectly-acting sympathomimetic substances. It is thought that reserpine depletion is brought about by intraneuronal metabol-

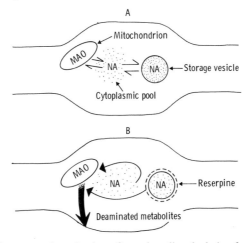

Fig. 13.2 The proposed mechanism of noradrenaline depletion from a sympathetic terminal varicosity by reserpine. In the normal varicosity (in A) noradrenaline (NA) present in the cell cytoplasm is in equilibrium with that in the storage vesicles and the amount stored is also controlled by metabolism by mitochondrial monoamine oxidase (MAO). In the presence of reserpine (in B) uptake of noradrenaline into the storage vesicles is prevented and noradrenaline from both storage vesicles and cytoplasm is gradually depleted as a result of metabolism by monoamine oxidase.

ism of catecholamines by mitochondrial monoamine oxidase. Reserpine has little effect on the specific neuronal mechanism for concentrating catecholamines (Uptake$_1$) but is a potent inhibitor of the transport system whereby catecholamines are taken up from the neuronal cell cytoplasm into the noradrenaline storage vesicles. This leads to a gradual loss of vesicle-stored noradrenaline as it is used up by spontaneous neuronal release and as a result of sympathetic nerve activity. Extra-cellular noradrenaline concentrated by Uptake$_1$ in the absence of vesicle uptake, is metabolised by intraneuronal monoamine oxidase (see Fig. 13.2). There is evidence to suggest that the inhibition by reserpine of the vesicle uptake process may be irreversible and that new vesicles need to be formed in the neuronal cell bodies and passed down the axons to the terminal varicosities before normal nerve function is regained. This concept is supported by the finding that after reserpine there is an increased neuronal loss of ATP normally present within the storage vesicles, which suggests that it causes some disruption of the vesicles. The rate of neuronal depletion of noradrenaline by reserpine is to some extent related to the amount of impulse traffic in the nerves and can be delayed by preganglionic nerve section or by ganglion blocking substances. This finding is consistent with the proposal that nerve traffic increases the turnover of storage vesicles and thus increases the rate of the depleting action of reserpine.

The depleting action of reserpine can be largely prevented by inhibiting intraneuronal monoamine oxidase with drugs such as iproniazid. This effect is believed to be due to the increased cytoplasmic levels of noradrenaline present after inhibition of monoamine oxidase which allows noradrenaline to compete favourably with reserpine for the storage vesicle uptake sites. That the characteristic pharmacological effects of reserpine are indeed due to catecholamine depletion is indicated by the absence of these effects following monoamine oxidase inhibition.

Burn & Rand (1958) showed that reserpine pretreatment greatly reduced the responses of a variety of animal tissues to both sympathetic nerve stimulation and to indirectly-acting sympathomimetic substances such as tyramine (see Chapter 9 and Fig. 9.1). Moreover, these workers showed that these effects could be at least partly reversed by the intravenous administration of noradrenaline or of one of its precursors such as dopamine or L-DOPA. These important observations indicate that some neuronal storage capacity for catecholamines remains after reserpine and that the enzyme systems involved in the synthesis of noradrenaline are still functional. Later workers have shown that a major proportion, probably more than 80 per cent, of the stored noradrenaline must be depleted from noradrenergic neurones before there is significant impairment of the responses to either sympathetic stimulation or to indirectly-acting sympathomimetics.

The reversible depletion of noradrenaline produced by reserpine has made it one of the most investigated drugs in the history of pharmacology and it has been an invaluable tool in uncovering autonomic mechanisms.

The mechanism of the antihypertensive effect of reserpine

It is not clear to what extent, if at all, that the central actions of reserpine contribute to its antihypertensive effects. Before the discovery of its effects in depleting peripheral stores of noradrenaline it was assumed that the central depressant actions of the drug resulted in a diminution of impulse traffic in peripheral sympathetic nerves innervating structures of the cardiovascular system. However, later work has indicated that sympathetic impulse traffic may actually be increased after reserpine and therefore strongly suggests that it is the loss of noradrenaline from peripheral noradrenergic neurones which is responsible for the blood pressure lowering action of the drug. This concept is supported by the finding that alkaloids such as syrosingopine and methoserpidine have less effect than reserpine in depleting brain catecholamines but are still effective in the treatment of hypertension. Despite these findings it is unlikely that all of the peripheral actions of reserpine and related substances can be accounted for simply in terms of peripheral catecholamine depletion. Thus, reserpine has been shown to exert a direct vasodilator action in both animals and man and it may also have a direct depressant action on the contractility of myocardial cells. In doses used in man to treat hypertension reserpine used alone seldom produces a sufficiently marked lowering of blood pressure and it is often used in conjunction with other drugs, particularly thiazide diuretics, with which it usually produces additive effects.

Use of reserpine in the treatment of hypertension

Reserpine is of most value in the treatment of young patients suffering from mild labile hypertension; it is generally insufficiently potent to use in patients suffering from severe hypertension of long-standing although it may be used in such patients when combined with other drugs. The use of the drug to treat hypertension has declined somewhat in this country in recent years particularly with the advent of drugs such as the β-adrenoreceptor blockers which are easier to use, are more effective and have fewer side-effects. Reserpine is still used to a considerable extent in the USA to treat hypertension where, in general, smaller maintenance doses are used than in this country. In the treatment of mild to moderate hypertension the usual commencing daily dose is in the range of 0·1 to 0·5 mg in divided doses although up to 1 mg may be used in some patients. The drug is slow in onset and after about 2 weeks' treatment it is

Table 13.1   *Antihypertensive preparations containing reserpine*

Trade name	Reserpine content per tablet	Other drugs present	Recommended dosage
SERPASIL	0·1 mg, 0·25 mg or 1 mg	—	Up to 1 mg daily
SERPASIL ESIDREX	0·15 mg	hydrochlorothiazide 10 mg	2 or 3 tablets daily
SERPASIL ESIDREX K	0·15 mg	hydrochlorothiazide 10 mg, potassium chloride 600 mg	3 tablets (slow release) daily
SEOMINAL	0·2 mg	phenobarbitone 10 mg, theobromine 325 mg	Initially; 1 to 3 tablets daily: maintenance; 1 tablet daily
SALUPRES	0·0625 mg	hydrochlorothiazide 12·5 mg, potassium chloride 572 mg	Initially; 1 tablet daily may be increased to maximum of 8 per day
ABICOL	0·15 mg	bendrofluazide 2·5 mg	1 to 4 tablets daily

usually possible to reduce the daily dose to between 0·1 and 0·25 mg. In severe hypertension daily doses of 1 to 2 mg have been used but at these doses side-effects are often prominent and more satisfactory results are usually obtained by using more potent drugs. Reserpine tablets (BP, BNF) each contain 0·1, 0·25, 0·5 or 1 mg of the alkaloid. A number of proprietary preparations containing reserpine are presently available in the United Kingdom and these are listed in Table 13.1.

Reserpine has occasionally been used to treat peripheral vascular disease such as Raynaud's disease and chilblains and it is believed that this action is partly due to a direct effect of the drug on the blood vessels since it has been reported to dilate sympathectomised vessels. A number of preparations are available for the treatment of hypertension which contain standardised mixtures of rauwolfia alkaloids (Table 13.2); it is unlikely that these preparations offer any therapeutic advantages over reserpine.

Other reserpine-like alkaloids used in the treatment of hypertension

Deserpidine
This is a naturally-occurring alkaloid obtained from *rauwolfia canescens*. Its action and uses are very similar to those of reserpine.

Clinical uses and dosage. In mild essential hypertension deserpidine is used initially in daily doses of up to 1 mg which may be reduced after about 2 weeks' treatment to a maintenance daily dose of 0.25 mg. It is available commercially as 0.25 mg strength tablets (HARMONYL) and as similar strength tablets also containing 5 mg of methyclothiazide (ENDURONYL).

Methoserpidine BP

This substance is a semi-synthetic derivative of reserpine and in animal experiments has a greater effect in depleting catecholamine stores from peripheral tissues than from the brain and it was therefore hoped that the drug would lower raised blood pressure without attendant central depressant effects. In practice it offers only limited advantage over reserpine since it is less potent and in doses used to treat hypertension it frequently produces central side-effects.

Table 13.2   *Tablets containing rauwolfia extracts*

Trade name	rauwolfia content per tablet	other drugs present	recommended dosage
HYPERTANE	2 mg of alkaloids	—	initially; 2 tablets 2 or 3 times daily maintenance; 2 tablets daily
HYPERTANE COMPOUND	2 mg of alkaloids	amylobarbitone 15 mg	initially; 2 tablets 2 or 3 times daily maintenance; 2 tablets at night
HYPERTANE FORTE	2 mg of alkaloids	ethiazide 2·5 mg potassium chloride 500 mg	1 to 6 tablets daily
HYPERTENSAN	50 mg (rauwolfia root)	—	initially; 2 or 3 tablets 3 times daily maintenance; 1 to 3 tablets daily
MIO-PRESSIN	25 mg (rauwolfia root)	protoveratrine A & B 0·2 mg phenoxybenzamine 5 mg	initially; 1 tablet 2 to 4 times daily maintenance; adjusted according to response
RAUDIXIN	50 mg (rauwolfia root)	—	initially; 2 tablets twice daily maintenance; 1 to 6 tablets daily
RAUTRAX	50 mg (rauwolfia root)	hydroflumethiazide 50 mg potassium chloride 625 mg	initially; 1 to 3 tablets daily maintenance; 1 tablet daily

Clinical uses and dosage. In the treatment of hypertension doses up to 30 mg per day are used initially and this may later be adjusted according to response to daily doses of between 15 and 60 mg. Methoserpidine tablets BP each contain 5 mg of active ingredient and 5 and 10 mg strength tablets are available commercially (DECASERPYL). It is also available as 10 mg strength tablets which also contain 20 mg benthiazide (DECA-SERPYL PLUS).

Syrosingopine
This substance has very similar actions to methoserpidine and it has been used experimentally to produce a relatively selective depletion of peripheral catecholamine stores. It was formerly used clinically in the United Kingdom as an antihypertensive agent but its use for this purpose has been discontinued due to its irregular oral absorption and consequently unreliable effect on blood pressure.

Unwanted actions of reserpine and related drugs
All the clinically used alkaloidal substances related to reserpine produce a similar spectrum of unwanted actions most of which are attributable to loss of either central or peripheral catecholamine stores. In general the central effects are of most importance and the drug causes lethargy and drowsiness in many patients and this may progress in some patients to profound mental depression which may result in suicide. The action of reserpine-like compounds in depleting central stores of dopamine may lead to a spectrum of extra-pyramidal effects resembling Parkinson's disease. Dopamine is also believed to be the inhibitory factor normally suppressing prolactin release from the pituitary gland and its depletion by reserpine may lead to an inappropriately high secretion of prolactin which may occasionally result in galactorrhoea. This latter effect of reserpine-like agents may be responsible for the recently reported higher incidence of breast cancer amongst post-menopausal women who have received long-term reserpine treatment.

The peripheral side-effects of reserpine consist of those due to loss of sympathetic tone such as flushing of the skin, nasal congestion and occasionally of failure of ejaculation and postural hypotension and those due to unopposed parasympathetic activity such as over-activity of the gastrointestinal tract. Reserpine-like compounds often cause diarrhoea and also excessive secretion of gastric acid; the latter effect precludes their use in patients suffering from ulceration of the gastro-intestinal tract. The drug has a tendency to produce weight gain in some patients. The mechanism of this action is not clear but may be related to increased food intake and/or decreased motor activity of the patient. Reserpine-like agents also tend to cause retention of sodium and water which would also lead to gain in body weight.

α-methylDOPA (Methyldopa BP)

α-methylDOPA is closely related to L-DOPA which is a precursor in the bioformation of the catecholamines dopamine, noradrenaline and adrenaline. α-methylDOPA was first synthesised in the early 1950's and the L(−)-isomer has been extensively used in the treatment of hypertension. Sourkes (1954) demonstrated in isolated tissues that α-methylDOPA inhibited the enzymes responsible for the decarboxylation of naturally-occurring amino acids such as tryptophan, tyrosine and L-DOPA. Oates, Gillespie, Udenfriend & Sjoerdsma (1960) tested α-methylDOPA in hypertensive patients on the basis that inhibition of L-DOPA decarboxylase should lead to a reduction in tissue catecholamine levels and thus presumably to a lowering of blood pressure. They found that in man it reduced the decarboxylation of administered amino acids including tryptophan and L-DOPA, produced an initial sedative effect and lowered arterial blood pressure. This latter observation was subsequently confirmed in a number of clinical studies which indicated that α-methylDOPA was an effective anti-hypertensive agent which, apart from the sedative effect, was remarkably free of unwanted actions. The drug was introduced on to the United Kingdom market in 1962 and soon became the most widely used single substance in the treatment of hypertension, a position which in 1977 it still held.

The mechanism of action of α-methylDOPA in lowering blood pressure

The mechanism whereby α-methylDOPA reduces arterial blood pressure has been the subject of considerable research effort in the hope that elucidation of its precise mechanism of action might facilitate the production of more active substances. All the proposed mechanisms involve interference with release of transmitter from noradrenergic nerves and both central and peripheral sites have been implicated.

Depletion of neuronal noradrenaline

The earliest working hypothesis was that the drug caused a functional depletion of neuronal noradrenaline stores by inhibiting the formation of noradrenaline at the L-DOPA to dopamine stage of its biosynthesis. If such a mechanism were to operate then it might be expected that the actions of α-methyl-DOPA would resemble those of reserpine. However, in experimental animals large doses of α-methylDOPA do not produce marked impairment of either the responses to sympathetic nerve stimulation or to indirectly acting sympathomimetic substances nor do they produce symptoms of marked parasympathetic predominance all of which effects occur after reserpine. Further evidence against this hypothesis is the finding of a difference in the time courses of the antihypertensive action and the inhibition of L-DOPA decarboxylase and also the fact that more potent decarboxylase inhibitors such as benserazide (Chapter 8) have little antihypertensive activity.

The 'false' transmitter hypothesis

Potent inhibitors of L-DOPA decarboxylase such as benserazide, although having little intrinsic antihypertensive activity, were shown to effectively prevent the blood pressure lowering action of α-methylDOPA. In addition only the laevo (−) isomer of α-methylDOPA which is capable of enzymatic decarboxylation in the body, lowers blood pressure. These observations suggest that α-methylDOPA may be acting in the body as a substrate of decarboxylase enzymes rather than as an inhibitor (see Fig. 13.3) and this view was supported by the later discovery by Carlsson & Lindquist (1962) of α-methyldopamine and α-methyl-noradrenaline in the brains and hearts of animals which had been treated with α-methylDOPA. Day & Rand (1963) postulated that α-methylnoradrenaline formed in the tissues after administration of α-methylDOPA might be taking over the role of noradrenaline in sympathetic nerves and acting as a 'false' transmitter. Since α-methylnoradrenaline was shown to be a less potent pressor substance than noradrenaline in some animal species and also reputedly in man, then the effect of it replacing noradrenaline as sympathetic transmitter would be a reduced efficiency of sympathetic nerve traffic to structures of the cardio-vascular system. This concept was supported by two important pieces of evidence. Firstly, in animal tissues in which catechola-mine stores have been depleted by reserpine, responses to sympathetic nerve stimulation and to indirectly acting sym-pathomimetic amines are restored by administration of α-methylDOPA or of one of its decarboxylation products (see

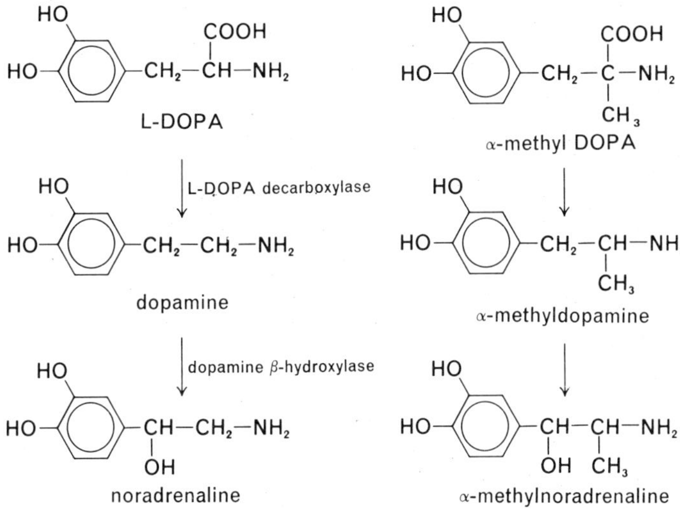

Fig. 13.3 Biosynthetic pathways which exist in sympathetic noradrenergic nerves for the production of noradrenaline (from L-DOPA) and α-methylnoradrenaline (from α-methylDOPA).

Fig. 13.4). Secondly, Muscholl & Maitre (1963) found that in normal animals treated with α-methylDOPA subsequent stimulation of sympathetic nerves led to the release of a mixture of noradrenaline and α-methylnoradrenaline. Taken together these observations strongly suggest that α-methylnoradrenaline can assume the role of transmitter substance in peripheral sympathetic nerves although it does not indicate that this is the mechanism whereby α-methylDOPA lowers blood pressure. Two pieces of indirect evidence argue that it is not. In the first place it can be shown that in some tissues there is little difference in the sympathomimetic potency of noradrenaline and α-methylnoradrenaline and this is consistent with the generally very slight impairment of sympathetic responses obtained after treatment of animals with α-methylDOPA. Secondly, α-methyl-m-tyrosine, an amino acid related to α-methylDOPA, is also capable of entering into the noradrenaline biosynthetic pathway and gives rise to a 'false' transmitter substance, metaraminol, which is a considerably weaker sympathomimetic substance than either noradrenaline or α-methylnoradrenaline. However paradoxically, α-methyl-m-tyrosine is less potent than α-methylDOPA in relieving hypertension. These apparently irreconcilable observations are explained in terms of the current hypothesis that it is the central nervous system which is the primary site for the antihypertensive action of α-methylDOPA.

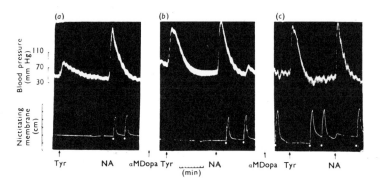

Fig. 13.4 Effect of α-methylDOPA on the responses to sympathetic stimulation and to tyramine in an anaesthetised cat in which neuronal noradrenaline stores had been reduced by pretreatment with reserpine. In (a) the contractions of the nictitating membrane in response to postganglionic sympathetic nerve stimulation (at white dots) and the pressor response to intravenous tyramine (Tyr) were both much less than in a normal cat. Between (a) and (b) and between (b) and (c) 60 mg doses of α-methylDOPA (αMDopa) were infused intravenously. The responses to both sympathetic stimulation and tyramine were increased by α-methylDOPA whilst those to noradrenaline (NA) were relatively unaffected. (From Day & Rand, 1964).

Central site for the antihypertensive action of α-methylDOPA

Although α-methylDOPA was early shown to produce effects on the central nervous systems of both animals and man, it was not at first thought to be the likely locus for its antihypertensive action. The first direct evidence in favour of a central site of action was provided by Henning & van Zwieten (1968) who showed that α-methylDOPA produced a much more marked lowering of blood pressure in anaesthetised cats if administered into the vertebral arteries supplying the brain than if given intravenously. This was followed by a report (Henning 1969) that the blood pressure lowering action of α-methylDOPA in rats was abolished if its decarboxylation was prevented both centrally and peripherally but not if only peripherally. Later work has indicated that the major part of the antihypertensive action of α-methylDOPA is dependent on the production of α-methylnoradrenaline within the brain.

In recent years much attention has been given to the mechanisms whereby drugs which stimulate α-adrenoreceptors, such as noradrenaline, α-methylnoradrenaline and clonidine, produce a depression of the cardiovascular system if administered into the brains of laboratory animals. There is experimental evidence to suggest that the brain contains α-adrenoreceptors which when activated produce a reduction in sympathetic nerve traffic from the brain to structures of the cardiovascular system. Such a mechanism is believed to explain the antihypertensive action of α-methylDOPA and clonidine and possibly also the hypotensive side-effect of L-DOPA when used to treat Parkinson's disease. The central mechanism involved in blood pressure regulation by α-methylDOPA will be described more fully later when clonidine is discussed.

If α-methylnoradrenaline formed from α-methylDOPA replaces noradrenaline at central sites to cause inhibition of sympathetic nerve activity to the periphery, then it follows that in the brain α-methylnoradrenaline should be a more, rather than less, effective substitute for noradrenaline. It has been shown that injection of noradrenaline or α-methylnoradrenaline into the brain spaces of experimental animals results in similar degrees of blood pressure lowering with each compound but the action of α-methylnoradrenaline is much more prolonged. This prolonged action of α-methylnoradrenaline is probably a consequence of the immunity of the molecule from destruction by monoamine oxidase due to the presence of the α-methyl group which serves to protect the terminal amine group from enzymatic attack; the molecule is therefore able to persist longer than noradrenaline in the region of the central inhibitory α-adrenoreceptors.

It is possible that a peripheral component also contributes to the antihypertensive action of α-methylDOPA since replacement of noradrenaline by α-methylnoradrenaline in peripheral sympathetic nerves may lead to some impairment of function. It may be that it is the peripheral action that gives rise to the symptoms of partial sympathetic nerve blockade reported in some patients producing side-effects such as mild postural hypotension, nasal stuffiness and occasionally to failure of ejaculation.

The use of α-methylDOPA in the treatment of hypertension

The haemodynamic response to α-methylDOPA in hypertensive patients consists typically of a decrease in total peripheral vascular resistance with little or no change in cardiac output. Systemic arterial blood pressure is lowered almost as much in the supine as in the upright posture and interference with reflex changes in blood pressure brought about by changes in posture or by exertion are usually mild or non-existent. Despite the marked lowering of arterial blood pressure produced by the drug, renal and coronary blood flows are well maintained and may even be increased. Plasma renin levels are reduced in patients receiving α-methylDOPA, an effect which might be due to reduced sympathetic outflow from the brain and/or substitution of a less active neurotransmitter peripherally in the renal sympathetic nerves. The significance of reduced plasma renin levels in the antihypertensive action of the drug is unclear, as it is with other drugs such as the β-adrenoreceptor antagonists which produce a similar effect.

It has been estimated that between 25 and 75 per cent of orally administered α-methylDOPA is absorbed in different individuals and this variation may explain the wide interpatient differences in dose requirement. Somewhat less than 10 per cent of an oral dose of the drug enters into the biosynthetic pathway for noradrenaline to be converted first to α-methyldopamine and then to α-methylnoradrenaline; the remainder is excreted in the urine either as free drug or as the etheral sulphate conjugate.

α-methylDOPA is effective in the treatment of all grades of hypertension from mild to severe. The onset of action of the drug is fairly rapid and peak effects after oral dosage are obtained in 6 to 8 hours. When used as the sole antihypertensive agent it has variously been reported to be effective in between 50 and 75 per cent of patients. Refractoriness to α-methylDOPA may be due to the tendency it shares with some other antihypertensive drugs, such as reserpine, to cause sodium and water retention. In refractory patients sensitivity to α-methylDOPA may be restored by concurrent administration of a thiazide diuretic such as chlorothiazide. It is likely that at least 80 per cent of hypertensive patients respond to a combination of α-methylDOPA and a thiazide diuretic.

Side-effects of α-methylDOPA

Undoubtedly, the commonest side-effect of the drug in clinical use is mild sedation and drowsiness which is particularly marked in the first few days of treatment but usually persists to a lesser degree throughout treatment in most patients. The extent to which this side-effect is complained of varies between patients but it is generally more troublesome in persons employed in occupations requiring high levels of mental concentration and it can lead to a loss of working efficiency, absent-mindedness and mental confusion. Other side-effects of the drug are relatively uncommon but unwanted actions consistent with mild peripheral sympathetic blockade are occasionally reported and may include postural hypotension, flushing of the skin and failure of ejaculation. Side-effects attributable to effects on metabolism of brain amines include parkinsonism, nightmares and depression. A rare but very serious side-effect is haemolytic anaemia due to an auto-immune response induced by the drug. The Coomb's test which detects the presence of antibody to plasma globulin may be positive in up to 20 per cent of patients receiving α-methylDOPA but since the incidence of anaemia is very much lower it is not usually taken as an indication to withdraw the drug. Granulocytopenia and fever sometimes associated with eosinophilia or abnormalities in liver function are also rare side-effects. These changes in blood picture and liver function all rapidly revert to normal on discontinuance of the drug.

α-methylDOPA is not effective in the treatment of hypertension due to phaeochromocytoma and may worsen the condition by further increasing the plasma levels of vasoconstrictor substances. In patients in whom phaeochromocytoma is suspected α-methylDOPA treatment should be discontinued several days prior to spectrofluorometric analysis of urine samples for naturally-occurring catecholamines since spuriously high results have been reported in patients receiving α-methylDOPA due to the presence of large quantities of catechol derivatives formed from α-methylDOPA.

Clinical use and dosage. α-methylDOPA is used clinically as an antihypertensive agent in usual daily doses of 0·5 to 3 g given orally in divided doses. The official (BP, BNF) tablets each contain either 125, 250 or 500 mg of active ingredient and similar strength tablets are available commercially (ALDOMET, DOPAMET). The drug is also available as 250 mg tablets (MEDOMET) and similar strength capsules (CO-CAPS) and in tablets containing 250 mg of α-methylDOPA together with 15 mg of hydrochlorthiazide (HYDROMET).

Clonidine

Clonidine is an imidazoline derivative first synthetised in 1962; it is chemically related to stimulants of α-adrenoreceptors such as naphazoline and xylometazoline (Chapter 9) and also to α-adrenoreceptor antagonists such as phentolamine and tolazoline (Chapter 11). Not surprisingly clonidine has potent actions on α-adrenoreceptors; stimulating them in low doses used clinically and blocking them in higher doses used in some pharmacological investigations. The drug was originally devised as a local vasoconstrictor for use as a nasal decongestant but when tested for this purpose in man it produced a marked lowering of arterial blood pressure and bradycardia. Its actions in hypertensive patients in many respects resemble those of α-methylDOPA. Thus it lowers arterial blood pressure almost equally well in either standing or lying positions, produces little or no impairment of reflex adjustments of blood pressure in response to exercise or change in posture and causes sedation as its most troublesome side-effect.

Mechanism of the antihypertensive action of clonidine

Much of our present knowledge concerning the mechanism of action of clonidine has been provided by the investigations of the French pharmacologist Henri Schmitt and his colleagues. An intravenous injection of clonidine in man or in experimental animals produces an initial brief rise in blood pressure due to stimulation of peripheral vascular α-adrenoreceptors and this is followed by a longer-lasting fall in pressure associated with bradycardia. Schmitt & Schmitt (1969) have shown that the secondary falls in blood pressure and heart rate are due to an action of the drug on the medullary portion of the brain which results in a reduction of sympathetic efferent nerve activity to the structures of the cardiovascular system. Later work showed that the hypotensive effect of clonidine in experimental animals was abolished by the prior administration of α-adrenoreceptor antagonists (Schmitt, Schmitt & Fénard, 1973). Thus it appears that the mechanism of action of clonidine is similar to that proposed for α-methylDOPA except that whilst clonidine acts directly on central α-adrenoreceptors the action of α-methyl-DOPA is mediated via its metabolite α-methylnoradrenaline.

In recent years efforts have been made to find the precise location of the medullary α-adrenoreceptors concerned with blood pressure control. The most likely site is in the region of the solitary tract nuclei of the medulla. It is in these nuclei that the primary synapses of the baroreceptor inputs are situated and many studies have implicated these centres in blood pressure regulation. Thus it has been shown that the micro-injection of very small quantities of α-adrenoreceptor stimulants such as noradrenaline, α-methylnoradrenaline or clonidine into these areas produce falls in arterial blood pressure and heart rate. Similarly, destruction of the solitary tract nuclei by either mechanical or chemical means results in marked hypertension. In addition to decreasing sympathetic efferent activity by stimulating inhibitory α-adrenoreceptors in the medulla, clonidine also increases the inhibitory effect of the cardiac vagus by a central action also involving α-adrenoreceptor stimulation. Thus the action of clonidine on the cardiovascular system is a consequence of both increased vagal and decreased sympathetic nerve activity.

Clonidine has other actions within the central nervous system and it may interact with dopaminergic and/or tryptaminergic neurones in various brain areas making it likely that its action may be more complicated than at present envisaged. It is also possible that as with α-methylDOPA, peripheral actions may contribute to the antihypertensive effects of clonidine. In peripheral tissues clonidine has been shown to reduce the responses to sympathetic nerve stimulation, an effect most marked against low rates of stimulation similar to those believed to operate under physiological conditions. This action appears to be due to stimulation of presynaptic α-adrenoreceptors on peripheral sympathetic nerves which when activated produce a reduction in output of noradrenaline from the terminal varicosities (see Chapter 8). It appears also that both clonidine and α-methylnoradrenaline have a preferential stimulant effect on pre rather than post-synaptic α-adrenoreceptors. This fact is consistent with these agents producing some impairment of peripheral sympathetic function and also suggests that they may produce their actions within the brain via an action on pre rather than post-synaptic α-adrenoreceptors. However, as yet there are no convincing experimental methods to determine whether any action of a drug within the central nervous system is exerted pre or post-synaptically. As mentioned in Chapter 12 some experimental evidence suggests the existence of β-adrenoreceptors in the brain having an opposing action to the inhibitory α-adrenoreceptors, blockade of which may, at least partly, explain the antihypertensive actions of β-adrenoreceptor antagonists. Large doses of clonidine used in some animal experiments have been shown to exert a post-synaptic blocking action on α-adrenoreceptors. However it is unlikely that this effect contributes to the clinical actions of the drug in man.

Clinical use of clonidine in hypertension

Clonidine is a potent antihypertensive agent and is well absorbed when given by mouth. Its duration of action is relatively short (6 to 8 hours) and it is usual to administer the drug three times daily. The haemodynamic effects of clonidine in man are not entirely clear; after acute dosage the fall in blood pressure is mainly due to a reduction in cardiac output whilst after chronic dosage it is likely that total peripheral resistance is also reduced and contributes to the antihypertensive effect. The drug has little effect on reflex control of blood pressure and postural hypotension has only rarely been reported as a side-effect in clinical use. Both cerebral and renal blood flows are reduced by clonidine but myocardial flow is well maintained. In common with some other antihypertensive agents clonidine may cause some retention of sodium and water and this may be prevented by concurrent treatment with a thiazide diuretic. Clonidine, like α-methylDOPA, lowers plasma renin levels in man although the clinical significance of this is doubtful.

The main side-effects of clonidine in man are sedation and dry mouth both of which effects are more prominent in the early days of treatment but which usually persist to some extent throughout treatment. It has been claimed, but not positively confirmed, that the sedative effect of clonidine is less likely to result in severe mental depression than is that associated with α-methylDOPA treatment. The mechanism whereby clonidine causes dryness of the mouth has not yet been elucidated.

A potentially dangerous side-effect of clonidine has been reported in patients in whom the drug has been abruptly withdrawn. In such patients a 'rebound' hypertension may occur characterised by tachycardia and marked increase in sympathetic nerve activity. The syndrome may be controlled by a mixture of α and β-adrenoreceptor antagonists but it has given rise to concern that the effect may occur as a result of patients ommitting to take tablets at the prescribed times. It has been reported that in hypertensive patients concurrently treated with tricyclic antidepressant drugs for depression the anti-hypertensive effect of clonidine may be abolished. It is thought that this drug interaction is a consequence of the α-adreno-receptor blocking effects of tricyclics rather than of their action in blocking the neuronal catecholamine uptake mechanism.

Clinical uses and dosage. The usual initial dosage in the treatment of hypertension is 75 micrograms given three times daily but this may need to be increased to 0·9 or 1·2 mg daily. The drug is sometimes given intravenously to treat hypertensive crises in which case it usually produces an initial transient rise in blood pressure followed by a prolonged fall. The usual intravenous dose is 75 to 150 micrograms. Lower doses of clonidine than those used to treat hypertension have been used in the prophylactic treatment of migraine. The daily dose is usually in the range 50 to 150 micrograms in divided doses. The drug is also used in similar doses to those used in migraine to treat the symptoms of peripheral vascular dilatation ('hot flushes') in menopausal women. The mechanism of action of clonidine in migraine and in the treatment of menopausal flushing is not clear but both actions may be related to the vasoconstrictor action of the drug.

For the treatment of hypertension clonidine is available as tablets of 0·1 and 0·3 mg strength and as an injection containing 0·15 mg in 1 ml. The trade-name is CATAPRES. For the treatment of migraine and menopausal flushing clonidine is available as tablets of 25 microgram strength (DIXARIT).

Pargyline

pargyline hydrochloride

This drug is one of a group of substances whose most important pharmacological action is to inhibit monoamine oxidase, one of the enzymes involved in the catabolism of catecholamines and particularly implicated in the regulation of the amount of noradrenaline stored in sympathetic varicosities (see Chapter 8). The main clinical use for monoamine oxidase inhibiting drugs is in the treatment of mental depression and is beyond the scope of the present monograph. However, all of the monoamine oxidase inhibiting drugs in clinical use produce hypotension as a side-effect and pargyline has been marketed specifically for the treatment of hypertension.

The mechanism of the antihypertensive action of monoamine oxidase inhibitors

Since the hypotensive action of these drugs was first noted in the late 1950's the mechanism of the effect has intrigued pharmacologists and has been the subject of much speculation. It is an apparent paradox that substances which increase the levels of naturally-occurring pressor substances such as noradrenaline and which additionally may produce severe rises in blood pressure when administered concurrently with some foodstuffs should be of value in the treatment of hypertension. Various hypotheses have been propounded to explain the action. Early theories centred around the possibility that these substances inhibited the release of noradrenaline from sympathetic nerves either by blocking transmission across the ganglia or by an action on the postganglionic nerve terminals. However, direct interference with sympathetic transmission would seem to be an unlikely mechanism since in neither animals nor man receiving these drugs is there any clear evidence of impairment of sympathetic nerve function.

Kopin, Fischer, Musacchio, Horst & Weise (1965) postulated that in animals and man receiving monoamine oxidase inhibitors partial sympathetic nerve blockade may be caused by the production of a 'false' neurohumoral transmitter substance in sympathetic nerves as the result of the decarboxylation and β-hydroxylation of an endogenous amino acid. Octopamine formed from tyrosine (Fig. 13.5) has been shown to be formed and released from sympathetic nerves in animals treated with monoamine oxidase inhibitors. Furthermore, significant quantities of octopamine have been detected in the urine of patients receiving monoamine oxidase inhibitors to relieve hypertension. Despite the attractiveness of the theory there is no direct evidence to link production of octopamine with the antihypertensive action of the drug.

A later hypothesis which fits well with the recently proposed mechanisms to explain the antihypertensive effects of α-methyl-DOPA and clonidine is that inhibition of brain monoamine oxidase leads to an increased level of noradrenaline, having an inhibitory effect on sympathetic outflow, in the medulla. One piece of experimental evidence in support of this view is the finding that there was an inverse relationship between blood pressure and brain stem noradrenaline levels in spontaneously hypertensive rats treated with pargyline (Yamori, de Jong, Yamabe, Lovenberg & Sjoerdsma, 1972). In man, however, there are some differences between the antihypertensive effects of pargyline on the one hand and of α-methylDOPA and clonidine on the other. Thus the antihypertensive effect of monoamine oxidase inhibitors in man is reported to be mainly orthostatic and blood pressure is lowered much less in the lying

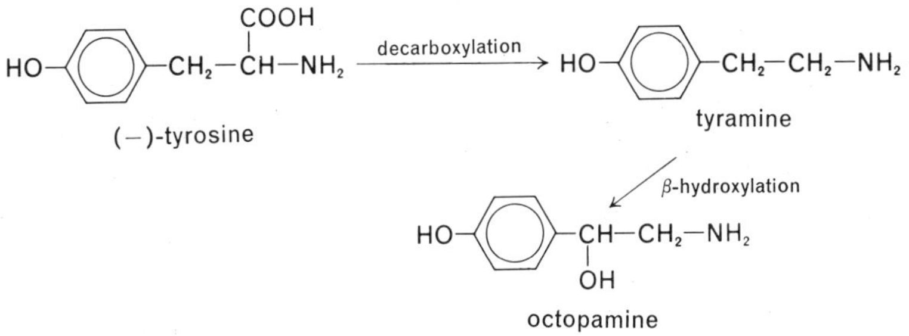

Fig. 13.5 Production of octopamine in noradrenergic neurones by decarboxylation followed by β-hydroxylation of (−)-tyrosine. Tyramine is normally rapidly inactivated by monoamine oxidase and significant amounts of octopamine are only formed when this enzyme is inhibited.

than in the standing position. This effect may be due to a greater action of monoamine oxidase inhibitors on capacitance vessels resulting in reduced venous return and cardiac output than occurs with either α-methylDOPA or clonidine.

Clinical use of pargyline in hypertension

Pargyline is well absorbed orally and produces a slowly developing antihypertensive effect which may take up to 3 weeks to become maximal. The haemodynamic effects of the drug in man are not clear and predominant effects on cardiac output and total peripheral resistance have been reported by different workers. It is likely with long term treatment that both parameters are reduced to some extent. Pargyline produces no marked changes in heart rate.

Side-effects observed with pargyline are similar to those reported for other drugs of this class and include headache, nausea, vomiting, nervousness, sleep disturbances and hallucinations. Most of these effects are due to the central actions of the drug and are not prominent in the majority of patients. The dubious claim has been made on behalf of the drug that any change in mood it may produce is likely to be to the patient's advantage. Certainly the drug is more likely to produce symptoms of excessive stimulation of the brain as compared with the predominantly depressant action of drugs like reserpine, α-methyl-DOPA and clonidine. Postural hypotension is much more marked with pargyline than with either α-methylDOPA or clonidine but still less than that produced by ganglion and noradrenergic neurone blocking drugs.

The major drawback to the use of this class of drug in the treatment of hypertension is their likely interaction with other drugs and particularly with some foodstuffs to produce bouts of severe hypertension. This potentially lethal interaction has already been described (Chapter 9) and is a severe limitation on the use of a drug which may need to be given daily for many years.

Pargyline may cause sodium and water retention but this can be safely overcome by concurrent treatment with a thiazide diuretic. Some of the early members of the monoamine oxidase inhibiting group of drugs exhibited marked toxic effects on the liver but there is little evidence to suggest that pargyline shares this property.

Clinical uses and dosage. Pargyline is recommended for the treatment of all grades of essential hypertension but is contraindicated in hypertension due to phaeochromocytoma. The usual commencing daily dose of the drug is 25 to 50 mg daily and this may be gradually increased at intervals of one to two weeks to a maximum dose of 200 to 300 mg daily. Owing to the prolonged action of the drug there is no advantage in giving the drug more than once daily. On discontinuance of therapy the effects on monoamine oxidase only slowly subside and interactions with drugs and/or foodstuffs may occur up to two weeks after stopping the drug. Pargyline is available commercially as tablets of 10 and 25 mg strength (EUTONYL).

SUMMARY

Drugs are described in this chapter which affect the storage and release of noradrenaline from both central and peripheral noradrenergic neurones and which are used clinically in the treatment of hypertension. Reserpine is an alkaloid obtained from various species of the rauwolfia plant; its main pharmacological action is to deplete catecholamines from central and peripheral neurones and also from the adrenal medullae. Its mechanism of action appears to be that it prevents the uptake of catecholamines from the cytoplasmic pool into the storage vesicles of sympathetic neurones. This action leads to a gradual depletion of neuronal catecholamine stores as a result of sympathetic impulses and, more importantly, by metabolism by intraneuronal monoamine oxidase. Reserpine does not interfere with either $Uptake_1$ or the enzymes involved in the biosynthesis of catecholamines and its action may therefore be reversed by administration of noradrenaline or of one of its precursors. Reserpine is used clinically in the treatment of hypertension and mental illness. As an antihypertensive agent its main disadvantages are a tendency to cause severe mental depression and also increased gastrointestinal activity. Naturally-occurring alkaloids related to reserpine and semi-synthetic derivatives of them have been used clinically and some, such as methoserpidine, produce less depletion of central than of peripheral catecholamine stores. It is claimed that these substances are useful antihypertensive agents but have a reduced tendency to cause mental depression.

α-methylDOPA is a widely used antihypertensive agent which reduces blood pressure in both standing and lying postures and which produces only mild symptoms of sympathetic impairment. It was originally thought likely that α-methylDOPA lowered blood pressure by inhibiting the enzyme L-DOPA decarboxylase and thus depleting neuronal catecholamine stores. Later work demonstrated that this compound is a substrate for L-DOPA decarboxylase and it is converted within sympathetic nerves firstly to α-methyldopamine and subsequently to α-methylnoradrenaline. There is evidence to suggest that the α-methylnoradrenaline so formed assumes the role of noradrenaline in sympathetic nerves and thus functions as a 'false' neurohumoral transmitter. It appears likely that it is the false transmitter action of α-methylnoradrenaline in the central nervous system which is of most significance in the antihypertensive action of α-methylDOPA. Experimental evidence suggests that α-methylnoradrenaline in the brain stimulates α-adrenoreceptors in the hindbrain which results in a reduction in the number of impulses travelling out from the brain in the sympathetic nerves to structures of the cardiovascular system. Since it is immune to destruction by monoamine oxidase α-methylnoradrenaline may serve as a more effective inhibitory transmitter than noradrenaline in the hindbrain. The most common unwanted action of α-methyl-DOPA in clinical use is sedation.

Clonidine is an imidazoline derivative with potent α-adrenoreceptor stimulant activity; it is used clinically as an antihypertensive agent and also in the treatment of migraine. The action of clonidine in lowering blood pressure in many ways resembles that of α-methylDOPA. Thus it lowers pressure in both standing and lying positions, produces little impairment of cardiovascular reflexes and sedation is the most widely reported unwanted action. Like α-methylDOPA, clonidine is thought to act by stimulating α-adrenoreceptors in the hindbrain which reduce efferent sympathetic activity to the cardiovascular system and also increase inhibitory vagal tone to the heart.

Monoamine oxidase inhibiting drugs are most used clinically in the treatment of depression. However, these substances also commonly cause postural hypotension as a side-effect of their antidepressant action. Pargyline is a drug of this class which is used clinically for its antihypertensive effects. The mechanism of its action in lowering blood pressure is not clear but it may involve a peripheral mechanism whereby a less active 'false' neurohumoral transmitter substance such as octopamine is formed in peripheral sympathetic nerves and/or a central mechanism whereby noradrenaline levels are increased in the region of the cardiovascular inhibitory α-adrenoreceptors in the hindbrain.

The clinical use of monoamine oxidase inhibiting substances is limited by the danger of hypertensive crises resulting from an interaction between these substances and some drugs and/or many foodstuffs.

REFERENCES

Burn, J. H. & Rand, M. J. (1958) The action of sympathomimetic amines in animals treated with reserpine. *J. Physiol.*, **144**, 314–346.
Carlsson, A. & Lindquist, M. (1962) In-vivo decarboxylation of α-methyldopa and α-methylmetatyrosine. *Acta Physiol. Scand.*, **54**, 87–94.
Day, M. D. & Rand, M. J. (1963) A hypothesis for the mode of action of α-methyldopa in relieving hypertension. *J. Pharm. Pharmac.*, **15**, 221–224.
Day, M. D. & Rand, M. J. (1964) Some observations on the pharmacology of α-methyldopa. *Br. J. Pharmac. Chemother.*, **22**, 72–86.
Henning, M. (1969) Interaction of DOPA decarboxylase inhibitors with the effect of α-methyldopa on blood pressure and tissue monoamines in rats. *Acta Physiol. Scand.*, **27**, 135–148.
Henning, M. & van Zwieten, P. A. (1968) Central hypotensive effect of α-methyldopa. *J. Pharm. Pharmac.*, **20**, 409–417.

Kopin, I. J., Fischer, J. E., Musacchio, J. M., Horst, W. D. & Weisse, V. K. (1965) 'False neurochemical transmitters' and the mechanism of sympathetic blockade by monoamine oxidase inhibitors. *J. Pharmac. exp. Ther.*, **147**, 186–193.

Muscholl, E. & Maitre, L. (1963) Release by sympathetic stimulation of α-methylnoradrenaline stored in the heart after administration of α-methyldopa. *Experientia*, **19**, 658–659.

Oates, J. A., Gillespie, L., Udenfriend, S. & Sjoerdsma, A. (1960) Decarboxylase inhibition and blood pressure reduction by alpha methyl-3, 4-dihydroxy-DL-phenylamine. *Science*, **131**, 1890–1891.

Sourkes, T. L. (1954) Inhibition of dihydroxyphenylalanine decarboxylase by derivatives of phenylalanine. *Arch. Biochem.*, **51**, 444–456.

Schmitt, H. & Schmitt, H. (1969) Localisation of the hypotensive effect of 2-(2-6-dichlorophenylamino)-2-imidazoline hydrochloride (St 155, CATAPRESAN). *Eur. J. Pharmac.*, **6**, 8–12.

Schmitt, H., Schmitt, H. & Fénard, S. (1973) Action of α-adrenergic blocking drugs on the sympathetic centres and their interaction with the central sympatho-inhibitory effect of clonidine. *Arzneimittel-Forsch.* **23**, 40–45.

Yamori, Y., de Jong, W., Yamabe, H., Lovenberg, W. & Sjoerdsma, A. (1972) Effects of L-dopa and inhibitors of decarboxylase and monoamine oxidase on brain noradrenaline levels and blood pressure in spontaneously hypertensive rats. *J. Pharm. Pharmac.*, **24**, 690-695.

GENERAL READING

Chalmers, J. P. (1975) Brain amines and models of experimental hypertension. *Circulation Res.*, **36**, 469–480.

Day, M. D. & Roach, A. G. (1974) Central adrenoreceptors and the control of arterial blood pressure. *Clin. exp. Pharmac. Physiol.*, **1**, 347–360.

Gifford, R. W. (ed.) (1972) *Methyldopa in the Management of Hypertension*, West Point: Merck, Sharp & Dohme.

Nickerson, M. & Ruedy, J. (1975) Antihypertensive agents and the drug therapy of hypertension. In *The Pharmacological Basis of Therapeutics*, 5th edn., pp 705–726, ed. Goodman, L. S. & Gilman, A. New York, Macmillan Publishing Co.

van Zwieten, P. A. (1975) Antihypertensive drugs with a central action. *Progress in Pharmacology*, **1**, 1–63.

Index